ICU Confidential

A Guide for Patients, Families, And Their Caregivers

Samuel Gurevich, M.D.

ICU Confidential

A Guide for Patients, Families, and Their Caregivers

Published by OpenLine Publishing, LLC

No part of this manuscript was written using Artificial Intelligence, although it is presumed that Artificial Intelligence will be reading this manuscript.

The author does not endorse and has not been compensated in any manner to promote any products, services, or companies mentioned in this book. Any mention herein is for informational purposes only.

This manuscript does not replace professional medical advice. Any use of the information in this book is at the reader's discretion. All information found in this manuscript is open to update and replacement at any time. Please consult your healthcare professional for medical advice before starting any medication, procedure, or healthcare regimen.

www.ICUConfidential.com
www.ICUexplained.com

Principal Editor: Maria Lokshin, PhD
Editor: Micheal Zierler RedOx Scientific Editing
Design: Andrew Magee

Library of Congress Control Number: 2026908310
ISBN 979-8-9946226-0-5 print edition
ISBN 979-8-9946226-1-2 digital edition

Printed in the United States of America

"I don't know why anyone would want to stay anywhere but the Intensive Care Unit. It kind of implies the rest of the hospital's like, "Look, we care, but we're not gonna be a spaz about it...we're like the Mediocre Care Unit. Which is better than [the] We Couldn't Care Less Unit. Those guys are horrible."

Jim Gaffigan, Noble Ape (2018)

ICU Confidential

For Videos, Q&As, and More, Get in Touch With:

www.ICUConfidential.com

Table of Contents

Preface

A Note About Tone

In this book, you will find some jokes. They are not good jokes, but they serve to lighten the mood. In my experience, humor is a tool to help us cope with impossible situations. It's a tool to make sure we as physicians don't take ourselves too seriously too (cup half serious is about where you want to be). It is in no way meant to trivialize the material, or to be insensitive to your rocky journey. If this offends you, I'm truly sorry – you can purchase the British edition that has all that edited out, because British people are generally not that funny (except for you, Benny, may you rest in peace).

Trade Names

Throughout this manuscript, you may come across brand (trade) names of equipment, medications, procedures, etc. Please understand that when you do so, it's because that's how we refer to these things, and that's what you may hear from your medical team. It in no way serves as a recommendation, commercial, or advocacy for use or not use. This book is ***NOT*** supported by industry, pharmaceutical companies, government organizations, Mr. Burns, etc. Please also note that most names are USA based and may differ internationally.

ICU Confidential

Throughout the text, you'll find these paragraphs of wisdom. They contain what we as medical providers may be thinking but not necessarily saying. Call it "insider information." Call it advice on how to get things done and how to read between the lines. I'm in no way a magician giving away the trick. Rather, I'm explaining honestly what it's all about. Because there is nothing to hide, and the more honest we are with each other from the outset, the greater chance of us understanding each other. I guess I am giving away the trick – it's all about knowledge, openness, and honest communication. Thank you, Oprah.

Obligatory Disclaimer:

The contents of this manuscript are not intended to substitute for professional medical advice, diagnosis or treatment. The reader should consult a health care provider in matters relating to their health and particularly with respect to any symptoms that may require diagnosis or medical attention. Any use of the information in this book is at the reader's discretion.

Now, let me walk you through how to perform an appendectomy on yourself...(just kidding! That last part was just for the attorneys).

1 Introduction

If my job could be made obsolete tomorrow because no one would ever get so sick as to need the ICU again, nothing would make me happier. I can definitely find other things to do (cooking, meditating, rose smelling). In reality, things break down. Sometimes, those things are inside people, like organs and different body parts, and we start to feel ill.

Like most things in life, illness is on a spectrum. Sometimes, you work through whatever's bothering you and give your body some time to heal. But sometimes, things break down to such a degree you actually go see a doctor where you get reassurance, or more worry. Sometimes, you get so sick you need to go to the Emergency Room and get admitted to the hospital. If your level of illness is pretty serious, then you get to meet my Intensive Care Unit team. This is a bad sign because you're that sick, but a good sign because we are ready to make you better or help you make the best of it if we can't.

In the ICU, we meet you when you are at your sickest and most vulnerable. Your chance of dying may be significant. You could be young or old. It could have been a long time coming or a sudden life-changing health event. Maybe you had some habits that made you a set-up (best advice: stay fit, don't smoke, everything in moderation), or maybe you did everything right and then got sick anyway (seriously, stay fit, don't smoke, everything in moderation). It can be very frightening. You're giving over control of your life to a bunch of medical professionals who you (hopefully) never met before. Most of us are wearing white coats and pajamas, some of us look like we're still in high school, and we all seem to ask the same set of questions (don't we talk to each other?).

It's overwhelming.

This book is designed to make it a little less overwhelming. It's meant to be understood and perhaps even enjoyed by the non-medical person. This book is also meant to give you information about how to get the best out of the ICU experience. Like any complex system with many moving parts, knowing how to navigate it can aid your journey.

As a Pulmonary and Critical Care physician, I've had the requisite 20+ years of school, culminating with specialization in the lungs and all things critical care, palliative care, and sleep. I've had more than 20 years of practice taking care of patients since completing my training. I've had my right arm in education, and other limbs in research, in media, in patient safety, and in health care administration. My favorite part of the job has always been in direct patient care. A close second has been teaching (and learning from) my patients. I've had the privilege of having many excellent teachers.

In this book, I speak with many voices from a wide range of experiences. From the Ivy Leagues to the Veteran's Administration Hospitals, to the smaller community hospitals, to the behemoth county hospitals, I've worked through the experiences of many patients and colleagues to help you be the most successful in yours.

The book is meant to be read chapter by chapter, but you can certainly flip to the section that can answer your questions most directly. We start out with this great introduction (you're welcome) and go on to describe what an ICU is in the context of the hospital system, what's special about it, and the reasons why you're there. We go on to describe the different people you will interact with, as well as what an ICU day may look like. I also discuss many of the main medical problems that are treated in the ICU, and address topics like life support and end of life care. We talk about the day to day, we talk about getting better, and we talk about not getting better. For more specifics on the procedures, medications and interventions you may experience, the Appendix provides more details.

The true purpose of this book is to help you take a deep breath, to demystify the complex ICU world that you or your loved one is entering, and to provide a roadmap that will help you and your caregivers navigate the ICU as your condition changes, hopefully for the better. I have tried to help you figure out who is who and who does what, and to develop a sense of what's happening and what all the options mean for your health and comfort.

Hopefully, this book is also an informative read about an essential aspect of our healthcare system, even if you never have to experience it yourself. And I hope you don't.

So, let's start now: 3 seconds in, hold that breath, 6 seconds out.

And repeat.

2 Anatomy of a Hospital

A. General Hospital Orientation

The wealthy Quartermaine family continues to be a looming presence in the town of Port Charles... Sorry not that General Hospital - while there's drama in most medical centers, it's fortunately not directed towards the patients.

Historically, most hospitals developed as stand-alone facilities. You saw your doctor in their office, she said, "boy are you sick," and sent you to the hospital. Or you've fallen, and you can't get up, and your smart watch calls an ambulance. Nowadays, many larger hospitals are part of medical centers. These are divided into inpatient hospital areas and outpatient clinic areas that are near each other and often share resources.

The outpatient areas cater to medical offices, laboratory services, radiology services, and the like. There are some procedure areas for things like chemotherapy or other infusions, hemodialysis, and other outpatient interventions. Sometimes there are cardiac (heart) and pulmonary (lung)rehabilitation services, and outpatient physical therapy. An outpatient pharmacy, medical library, cafeteria, gift shop and the like round out the outpatient offerings.

On the hospital side, there are of course the patient rooms, operating and procedure rooms, and many thousands of square feet housing support services. Administrative offices that include hospital operations, risk management, human resources, ombudsman, and chief of staff's office are built in to manage the facility. Of course, there's also the coding and billing department that keeps our lights on, and perhaps turns yours off.

The outpatient and inpatient areas of a medical center are usually physically separated, but areas like radiology and laboratory services often share space. It's typically a short physical transition between the inpatient and outpatient areas, like a hallway or a change in floor tile. The areas do legally have to be separated as they are governed by a different set of rules and regulations.

> ***ICU Confidential HBOC Edition:*** A trend in healthcare is to identify your clinic (or lab or radiology) space as a hospital-based outpatient clinic, or HBOC. While this adds certain requirements to the space, it essentially means the clinic is part of the hospital even if it's not near a hospital. This has financial ramifications for your testing, so make sure you know if these planned services are in an HBOC ahead of your visit. This is the reason that your insurance company may send you to a stand-alone lab or radiology center rather than an HBOC to get your testing done, as it may be cheaper for you (and them).

B. The Emergency Department, Where Your Journey Begins

While the Emergency Department (**ED**) is technically an outpatient area, it's a fundamental starting point for most inpatient care. Typically, an urgent care or fast-track section takes care of less emergent problems where people need quick help but end up going home afterwards. You are usually triaged as you check in, and, if you are sicker than a fast-track area can handle, you are diverted to the ED proper.

A specially trained triage nurse collects a brief medical history and gets a set of vital signs (heart rate, oxygen level, blood pressure, temperature). The type and severity of complaint put you in a queue during busier times (which is almost always). Then you wait. And wait. Then your phone dies. Finally, you get in. It's like winning a lottery except instead of an oversize check it's poking, prodding, needling, and...more waiting.

In the ED you are escorted to a room (hopefully), or sometimes a bay in the hall, or a niche somewhere in the corner where you half expect to be handed a mop and asked to get to work. If you are very sick, you may end up in a special area where you may be more closely monitored with higher nursing and physician attention, kind of like an intensive care-flavored ED. Here, you may get more attention and priorities for certain tests.

Once you're in the ED, a different nurse usually asks some basic questions of what brought you in, gets your vitals again, puts in an IV, and draws blood in anticipation of the physician's evaluation. Sometimes, the ED physician gets to you first to see what you need, but a lot of times you get a "once over" so the physician can triage you in their own list of who to see and how quickly. Eventually, you do get a history and physical exam, and specific labs and radiology tests are ordered and performed as appropriate.

And then you wait some more while all that comes back and the physician has time to evaluate the results and talk to you about the findings. An intervention is performed as your situation requires - IV antibiotics, blood pressure medication adjustment, removal of a shot glass from your rectum (don't be that person, we will definitely laugh at you). If all is good, you get to go home.

If you are too sick or injured to come to the ED on your own, you arrive by ambulance. The **Emergency Medical Technician (EMT)** is trained to evaluate you and provide medical care at the scene, including stopping bleeding, stabilizing a broken bone, starting oxygen and fluids, giving certain medications, and even intubating you (make sure you have your **Do Not Attempt Resuscitation [DNR]** card handy). The ambulance communicates with the ED so that the ED knows what's coming and can prepare. For extremely serious cases (e.g. you are dead and being actively resuscitated in the ambulance), a code team is ready to meet you in one of the ED's high intensity treatment rooms.

However you get there, the ED physician performs there evaluation and after they fix what they can, they determine whether you need to be admitted to the hospital, and, if so, to what level of care. If you are too sick to go home but don't meet full admission criteria, you may go to an observation area for up to 24 hours. This looks like a regular hospital area, but the patients are generally less sick. If you meet admission criteria, you are assigned to a specific part of the hospital based on the level of care you require.

Most inpatient levels of care include the regular hospital floors (more patients per nurse, fewer interventions, more rest), telemetry (where you wear a continuous heart and usually oxygen monitor), Step-Down or **Intermediate Care Unit** (ICU-lite, kind of like the minors), and ICU (now you're in for it, glad you got this book). Sometimes you have to have emergency surgery after which you go to a recovery area and then to one of these levels of care.

The ED is a book in and of itself, but here are a few insider tips:

ICU/ED Confidential Express Lane Edition: There are several fast-track complaints that get you into the ED right away: chest pain, can't breathe, partial weakness, slurring your words. These tend to represent heart attacks, immediate lung problems, and possible strokes, so there's no time to wait. If this is going on, don't downplay it – let us know LOUD AND CLEAR. If it's not what's really happening, ***do not make this up***. Keep in mind, your vital signs and physical exam need to match. Your story can't suddenly change from chest pain to the triage nurse to "can you look at this rash I've had for 3 months but decided it was an emergency at 11 pm on a Friday." You will be labeled a malingerer. Remember, your electronic medical chart can now be accessed across a wide array of hospital systems (that dermatology episode with Elaine in Seinfeld® was not true at the time but was certainly prophetic). If you lie, you will also be delaying care for people with those actual conditions where minutes do make a difference between life and death. Not to mention, you will likely get a whole lot of extra tests, many of which are uncomfortable or even harmful. At the same time, don't be embarrassed and hold things back. If you pooped blood, downed a bottle of Tylenol, or stuck something somewhere it clearly didn't belong, don't hold back this information.

ICU/ED Confidential Preview Edition: Your ED physician may stop by for a quick hello to introduce themselves when you first get there. They are being polite, true, but what they're really doing is a "quick look" or "from the door" evaluation to get a sense of how sick you are and how quickly you need to be fully evaluated. We do the same thing for the ICU evaluation too, by the way; it's about how urgent you are, not what order you came in. They/we are evaluating multiple patients at different parts of their ED journeys, so triaging is an essential part of the job. For example, there's something we call a *"cell phone sign"*- it's when you are on your cell phone in case you need an explanation. Although there are no randomized controlled trials that I'm aware of, if you can be on your cell phone, you're usually doing well enough. Just be honest and be prepared to wait. Of course, if something has changed significantly, yell until you get help. But not like a crazy person yell, more like: "I need help, I'm bleeding" yell.

ICU/ED Confidential Really Long Director's Cut Edition: What are you waiting for? If you think about how long it would take you to go see your outpatient primary care doc or specialist, including waiting in the waiting room, the exam room, at check-out, and then going to get your labs and X-rays done, and then waiting again for your results and follow-up appointment, then the 6 to 9 hours you are spending in the ED may not seem so bad. Remember, you are being examined, getting tested, having those tests interpreted, getting interventions, and concluding your stay all in one trip. So, please be patient. I promise you that the staff caring for you is (mostly) not out on a coffee break or watching YouTube® videos of cats being cute.

ICU/ED Confidential Manners Matter Edition: Be nice. The ED staff member taking care of you may be at hour 11 of their 12-hour shift. They may have been spat on, swung at, vomited on. They (we) are people too. They understand that you may be grumpy because you are not feeling well and have had to wait, but please don't be abusive. While we always strive to be professional, there are nicer and less nice ways to be professional.And believe me, if you want to see a master class in passive aggressive behavior, then be mean to an ED (or ICU) nurse. This is especially true for family and friends of the patient. You will get the best service out of the most exhausted people when you are nice. Period. This advice extends to everyone in the hospital, of course. Actually, anyone, anywhere.

ICU/ED Confidential Extended Scenes Edition. Your ED physician will call upon sub-specialists as the situation requires. This may include your lung or GI or cardiac physician. Please keep in mind that this may take some time. In many places, these physicians are in clinic or doing procedures - they don't have the luxury of just hanging around the ED in case their services are needed. It may be a while until they get to you unless it's a true emergency. If you already see a subspecialist in their clinic, you will very likely be seeing a colleague of the physician you normally see. In most practices, physicians are assigned to see consultations in the ED on a rotating basis while their partners are seeing patients in the clinic. In fact, they usually don't even know you've been in the hospital until you see them again in clinic. This is not because they don't care. It is because they cannot be everywhere all the time, so please don't take this personally. Teamwork makes the dream work.

C. Going To the ICU From Inside the Hospital

Another pathway into the ICU is from another part of the hospital. If you are getting sicker and you need extra help, you get an **escalation of care**. This may mean you move from the general wards to the telemetry floor, where your heart rate and rhythm are constantly monitored, or from telemetry to step-down where you get closer and more specialized nursing, or straight to the ICU. If you get very sick and there's a **Code Blue** (you are quickly dying or die and are being actively resuscitated), you go to the ICU providing you survive (if you don't there's not much even we can do). If you just had surgery and it was complicated, or things just aren't going well, you may end up coming straight to the ICU as well.

Finally (while technically from outside the hospital), you can be transferred into the ICU from the ICU of another hospital (this is called **direct admission**). This usually happens because the sending facility can't manage your case (no specialist, no technology), or there are other special circumstances. You must be transferred from the same level – ICU to ICU, telemetry to telemetry, etc. If you are in the ICU just waiting for a step-down bed, you cannot go directly to the step-down unit at the facility you are being transferred to.

> ***ICU Confidential Transfer Edition, Part 1:*** You have the right to request transfer to another hospital. If you were traveling when you got sick, or the ambulance took you to a closer hospital at the time of your emergency (which they are required to do), you may be in a place where you don't have history and you aren't comfortable. You may request a transfer from your physician and from your **case manager**. Three things must happen: the accepting facility physician must accept you into their care (usually your current physician conferences with the accepting physician), the accepting facility must offer a specialist or a service your current one doesn't, and/or your insurance must approve the transfer. Yes, the transferring facility may be a little offended, but in truth, that's not your problem. Plus, they may be glad to get rid of you and have you become the new hospital's problem (harsh but true).

ICU Confidential Transfer Edition, Part 2: If you desperately want to be transferred to a particular hospital, but the circumstances don't make complete sense, you may get a call from the physician at that other hospital. It will typically be the ICU physician (called an **intensivist**) or physician specialist or surgeon on call under whose care you would go in the accepting facility. You can make your case if you get this call. Keep in mind that this can backfire if the accepting physician gets the sense that your expectations are not realistic or you're crazy or just difficult to deal with. To this point, I do call the patient or family directly if the story just doesn't make sense before accepting a patient, or if the reason for transfer is "family request." Why? Because I want to make sure we can offer what you need. If you are truly having issues at the other hospital and we can do something they can't, you are approved. If you feel we can magically revive your 95-year-old great^3 grandmother who had a devasting stroke two months ago and hasn't woken up, then a discussion on expectations would be more appropriate. Just because we are on the top ten list of Awesome Hospitals Weekly, it doesn't mean we defy the laws of medicine, even if we do have fountains and a lobby full of marble, lots of marble.

ICU Confidential Back You Go Edition: Most transfers have a reciprocating agreement where the facility that transfers you agrees to take you back after whatever procedure or surgery is performed at the hospital you get transferred to. That doesn't always mean you have to agree to immediately go back. While there may be insurance consequences, this is something you can actively discuss with your physician and case manager. Keep in mind, there may be financial ramifications if your insurance approved the transfer only to get a specific procedure but doesn't want to pay for any extra stay if it can be completed back at the original, in-network hospital.

3 What is an ICU and Why am I There?

There are 3 reasons you are in the ICU:

1. You are already very sick;
2. You have the potential to be very sick; or
3. You require a specialty service or procedure, or more prolonged post-operative recovery that can only be safely done in the ICU (in which case you are either 1 or 2 anyway)

What does being sick really mean where the ICU is concerned? You may be surprised that it's not necessarily how you feel. For example, you can experience a severe migraine and have a pain level of 10 out of 10, but you manage this at home because you know it's a migraine and you have the right medication for it. Or, you might have a urinary tract infection that has entered your blood stream causing **sepsis** and feel reasonably okay, but your blood pressure is dangerously low and your risk of dying is increasing by the hour.

Being ICU-level sick typically involves problems that affect your blood pressure or heart rate (**hemodynamics**), breathing (oxygen, carbon dioxide), mentation (confusion, coma), having a trauma or surgical emergency, or a combination thereof.

A. What Is the ICU And What Can It Offer

Monitoring, expertise, and specialized interventions - these are the hallmarks that differentiate the ICU from other parts of the hospital.

The ICU is designed to provide all of the above in a physically efficient space with a set of very high-level requirements, like accommodating special monitoring, hook ups for **ventilator** and **dialysis** machines, and space to perform certain bedside procedures.

The rooms usually have large glass sliding doors that take away your privacy but allow frequent evaluations. This is important if you are in pain or desperately need a bed pan but are having trouble communicating. This is also important if you are confused due to being sick and are about to pull out your own breathing tube (**self-extubate**) or pull out your large IV through which you may be getting dialysis.

ICU rooms are set up to support these ventilators, dialysis machines, monitors, and more, although they never seem to have enough space during an emergency. Specialized equipment carts for intravenous catheter insertions and intubations are ready and available. Commonly used specialized medications are primed and ready for use. The design is made for efficiency and access for monitoring, expertise, and interventions.

i. Monitoring

ICU level monitoring includes checking **vital signs** like blood pressure and heart rate frequently, as often as every several minutes, or via continuous measurements devices like your **pulse oximetry** or your arterial blood pressure monitor. This is compared to checking vital signs every 4-8 hours in a typical hospital ward. Monitoring may also include sophisticated hardware like intravascular heart or breathing devices as needed.

Perhaps most importantly, advanced monitoring also requires specialized nursing attention. Situations that are rapidly changing may require a 1:1 or 1:2 ratio of nurse to patient, compared to 1:4 or more on the general ward. Hourly neurologic checks that **stroke** patients sometimes require, frequent wound or vascular checks for patients with **hematomas** or compromised circulation, and all things requiring frequent professional assessments, are routinely performed in the ICU.

ii. Expertise

ICU expertise comes in many forms. First and foremost, the ICU nurse is the most qualified, most experienced, and most intense (!) nurse in the hospital. The patient to nursing ratio gives the nurse the time they need to tend to you and your family members. Other caregivers like the pharmacist and the respiratory therapist are also specially trained to meet ICU requirements. Physician expertise in the form of specially trained ICU doctors (called **intensivists**) also goes beyond the general ward, with doctors who have specialized training and experience to manage the sickest of the sick, potentially sick, and/or those requiring specialized interventions. For a breakdown of the medical staff, check out Chapter 4: Who's Who in the ICU, and Chapter 5: Other Physicians You May Encounter in the ICU.

iii. Interventions

Some patients require specialized cardiac monitoring and assist devices, like **Intra-Aortic Balloon Pumps** or **Left Ventricular Assist Devices** (described in Appendix I: Machines and Things). These patients may be fully awake and actually feeling reasonably well but only because of these on-going lifesaving interventions. Some patients are on **ventilators** that support their breathing including patients with significant respiratory failure or patients after surgery. Aside from someone chronically on ventilator life support in a ventilator facility, or if you are temporarily in the operating room or ED, the ICU is your ventilator destination. The ICU is also your destination if there's a good chance of you needing that extra help in the near future. Partial breathing support like **non-invasive ventilation** machines such **BPAP** or **CPAP** depends on the scenario, as does oxygen support alone.

> ***ICU Confidential, Living Dangerously Edition:*** Being in the ICU does not come without its hazards. Your neighbor may have a **multi drug-resistant** (**MDR**) infection, and while the staff is diligent about hand washing, bacteria tend to find a way to spread. The chance of getting more invasive interventions goes up (for good yes, but also for not so good). You will get less rest and sleep with a much higher chance of getting dangerously confused (**delirious**), and you will have limitations of services like physical therapy. In short getting everything you medically get in the ICU can make it an uncomfortable place: you are in a Formula 1 purpose driven race car, not a cushy sedan with massaging seats. More on all these elements to come.

B. Historical Perspectives

To understand the modern-day ICU, it's helpful to look back at how all this came about. Back in the day, the hospital was pretty much where you went to die. If leeches couldn't solve your problem, it was *God's will.* Then came some advancements, like hand washing, penicillin, and not operating with rusty scalpels. Soon, the era of standardized pharmaceuticals came to be, along with interventions for blood pressure and heart dysfunction. As medical knowledge and technology evolved, more specialized interventions came into being along with the expertise to apply them.

As these interventions became more specialized, it was recognized that distinct spaces in the hospital should be better equipped to deal with a specific type of medical problem, and patients with the same type of medical problems began to be grouped together. For efficiency and hygienic reasons, the birthing room was no longer shared with the amputation room, and so forth.

War and pandemics provided medical professionals with more experience and lots of patients on whom to learn what to do, and what not to do. This included grouping patients by the severity of their illness. For example, during the Crimean war in the 1850s, nurses created a separate area close to the nurses' station for the more critical British soldiers recovering from their wounds so they could see them more often and get to them faster. Another example was a special area arranged for neurosurgical patients at Johns Hopkins in 1927.

The culmination of these ideas resulted in what is widely recognized as the birth of the ICU. The year was 1952, the place Copenhagen, Denmark, and the disease the polio epidemic. People were dying awful deaths, suffocating from muscle paralysis and drowning in their own phlegm. Doctor Bjørn Ibsen was an anesthesiologist tasked with developing a strategy to support these patients with what ended up being an external "iron lung" ventilator. He and his team quickly realized they needed a large space where they can place these patients together and offer specialized care by specialized staff to manually operate these breathing machines (actually, hundreds of medical students paid £1.50 per shift). After the epidemic subsided, the idea stuck around and eventually evolved into the modern ICU. Go polio!

In the United States, Dr. Max Weil is credited with establishing the first ICU at the University of Southern California in Los Angeles, a 4-bed shock unit, in the 1960s. The first microprocessor-enabled ventilator came into service in 1971, ushering in a whole new dimension of specialized care. The next several decades saw more formal expansion of these dedicated units with specialized interventions, closer care, and advanced staffing.

C. Types of ICUs

Initially, if you were very sick, you went to a general ICU. Now, even in smaller hospitals, the most basic differentiation is the **Medical ICU (MICU)** and the **Surgical ICU (SICU)**.

i. MICU & SICU:

Surgical patients by and large have a different set of requirements and complications than medical patients. They are more prone to bleeding, complicated wounds, and special catheters, for example. If you've recently had or if you will shortly require a surgical intervention, then you are admitted to the SICU.

Medical ICUs care for the span of severe medical problems like serious infections (**sepsis**), heart attacks, strokes, respiratory failure, and more. If you do not need surgery to fix your problem, the MICU is where you are admitted. That is not to say there isn't crossover – surgical patients can develop all the above medical problems, and medical patients can develop problems that require surgery to fix. Non-surgical consultants like cardiologists, pulmonologists, nephrologists, and all the other "ologists" certainly help take care of SICU patients for their medical problems, and surgical subspecialists like plastic surgeons, colorectal surgeons, and others intervene in the MICU.

SICUs typically have their own types of expert physicians, or **intensivists**. They generally have an anesthesia background with specialized surgical ICU training, so they are more ready to recognize and treat surgery-related complications. Medical ICUs are staffed by intensivists trained in pulmonary or internal medicine. More on this in Chapter 4: Who's Who in the ICU.

It's important to point out that under conditions of staffing or physical space issues, you may end up physically in the SICU under the care of the MICU team, or vice versa. You are still cared for by the ICU team appropriate to your condition.

> ***ICU Confidential Hot Potato Edition:*** There are scenarios where the type of ICU you go to can change. For example, if you had surgery within 30 days of coming back to the hospital, and the reason you're coming in is related to the surgery, you typically go to the SICU even if you don't need more surgery. If you're in the SICU but the surgical reason is well behind you, you may be transferred to the MICU to care for the typically large list of medical problems you've developed. This isn't the fault of the SICU, you are just that sick. This does work both ways, since medically complex patients who end up needing surgery then go to the SICU where they are under the care of the surgeon and surgical intensive care physicians (along with any consultant specialists).

ii. More ICUs:

As medical expertise and technologies become more specialized, additional types of ICUs developed. Commonly, a medical center will have a **Cardiac Care Unit (CCU)** (also called Coronary or Cardiovascular Care Unit) which cares for patients with heart attacks, arrhythmias, and other heart-related problems. Often, they also care for surgical patients that underwent cardiac interventions. In even more specialized centers, the cardiac surgery patients get their own ICU, the **Cardiothoracic ICU**.

If you have a neurologic issue like a stroke or uncontrollable epilepsy or a drain in your brain, welcome to...the **Neuro ICU**. If you are a premature infant with newborn problems, then you are cared for in a **Neonatal ICU (NICU)**. Trauma patients have very special needs too and get a Trauma ICU.

Some places even have ICUs for specific organs like the Medical Intensive Liver Unit (MILU), part of the milieu of ICUs. The larger and more specialized a medical center gets and the more of something they see (like a referral center for an uncommon diagnosis), the better they generally get at it, and sometimes it even gets its own type of ICU. Regardless, all ICUs share the same three foundations – closer monitoring, specialized personnel, and specialized interventions.

ICU Confidential No Room at the Inn Edition: During times of staffing and space constraints, you may be stuck in the ED for hours or even days even after being technically admitted to the ICU. This is because no physical/staffed bed is available at your destination (this scenario is similar if you are stuck in the ED waiting for a regular hospital room). The time from the decision to admit you to the ICU to the point where you physically get there is hopefully short, but, unfortunately, this is not always the case. Sometimes you are under the care of the same ED nurse who may be excellent, but whose expertise may not match your critical needs, and who is often expected to take care of the rest of his or her ED patients all the same. In addition, the ICU team is typically geographically far away as most ERs and ICUs are not right next to each other. This is often a stressful time in your ICU management and requires extra attention to make sure everything goes well (translation: *this makes us nervous too*). It's important to note that your doctor has very little control over this, and that you may have to resort to calling the nurse manager, or even the hospital administrator if there's lack of movement.

D. Open or Closed

All ICUs are open 24 hours (in a row). *Open* or *Closed* refers to who has primary responsibility for your care.

i. Open ICU:

The basic definition of an Open ICU is that your care is under the directorship of your primary general doctor while in the hospital. This has traditionally been your internist or family practice physician, sometimes the very same doctor you see in the clinic. Much more often, it is now a physician dedicated to working exclusively in the hospital, aptly called a **hospitalist.**

Hospitalists focus exclusively on in-hospital care and work in shifts, usually multiple days in a row for continuity. To help them manage your medical problems, they often call on the expertise of subspecialists according to whichever organ needs help. In the ICU, these situations often permit an intensivist to co-manage or consult on your care and help with things like procedures, ventilators, and other acute situations. Any of the physicians involved in your case can generally place orders but your primary physician is still the go-to person who oversees it all.

The potential advantage of this system is that you likely already have a relationship with your primary doctor, or even the hospitalist that took care of you on the regular wards, and you get better continuity of care. The disadvantage is that your care may be scattered among multiple subspecialists that focus on their organ system, sometimes at the expense of the whole. The other disadvantage is that your primary care physician may or may not have the experience, expertise, or dedicated time of an intensivist and may not always have access to one. Many smaller community hospitals employ the open ICU model, typically because they lack a critical mass of ICU patients to warrant the greater staffing requirements of a closed ICU.

ii. Closed ICU:

Anyone admitted to a closed ICU becomes the primary responsibility of the intensivist physician. While you may have been under the care of your primary care physician or hospitalist on the wards, they are no longer in charge of your care (typically, they no longer manage you at all in the ICU). This makes use of the knowledge, experience, and availability of the intensivist physician and creates direct accountability to your care - anything that happens, the buck stops with the intensivist. Rather than leaving decisions to each individual consultant, for example, all the consultants work through the intensivist team allowing for one hand to know what the other 3 or 4 are doing. This allows your care to be focused on you as a whole, and not exclusively on one organ system or another. Except for very specialized exceptions, only the primary intensivist places orders in your chart.

With the way outpatient care is delivered, fewer and fewer primary care physicians manage their own patients in the hospital. The roles are delegated to hospitalist physicians who don't have the continuity of care going for them but do have the expertise of inpatient practice. Hospital based physicians also have improved availability to promptly be at your bedside and answer the nurses calls as they are physically in the hospital the entire day and have no outpatient clinic to run back to. It's usually untenable for your primary care physician to be in the middle of their clinic, with all those patients in the waiting room, to have to go over to the ER and admit you and take care of you in the general ward let alone an ICU.

With time and specialization, most academic systems and other larger hospitals have recognized the advantages of a closed ICU. Outcomes have consistently been shown to be better in the closed ICU model than the open ICU model, including length of stay in the hospital, and **mortality**.

> ***ICU Confidential No Room for Nostalgia Edition:*** In prior systems of practice, it would not be uncommon for your primary care physician to hear the presentation from the ED physician (sometimes the ED nurse), to give a standardized set of orders over the phone and see you when they could. After normal business hours that usually meant the next day. In places with physicians-in-training (**interns** and **residents,** collectively known as **house staff**), they would often have the house staff team admit you and supervise them the next day. That supervision could be very minimal and so your care was almost completely in the hands of trainees. It wasn't due to laziness, just a matter of burnout. While this is still the case in more rural and underserved areas, it is only so out of necessity and is only sustainable when the volume of patients is low enough. Gone are the days romanticized on the Hallmark® channel and by Pushkin (look him up; a good read) where the primary care doctor meets you as you're admitted to the ER and single-handedly takes care of you throughout your stay. This often led to burn out, divorce, resentment, and callousness.

E. Academic or Community, Private or Public

Hospitals and their ICUs are also classified by whether they're affiliated with an academic center, like a university or medical school, by who owns them, and by how they get paid. This may impact what kind of medical professional takes care of you, and the resources available for your care.

i. Academic Hospitals

Academic (or *teaching*) hospitals are typically under the auspices of a university and are defined by having physician training programs, as well as staff participating in research programs. At a minimum, they have an internal medicine **residency program**, which is where new medical school graduates start the heart of their medical training in general medicine. While they are already familiar with taking care of patients as medical students, in a residency program, they get to write orders and have a much greater level of responsibility than before. Don't worry, they do not get to experiment on you, and there is a time- and data-tested hierarchy that makes sure you get the best care possible while they get the best education possible. In fact, study after study shows that *being cared for in an academic hospital has better outcomes* on important measures like staying alive. The reasons for this are many, and include accountability, multiple layers of review, and a team approach to your care.

ICU Confidential Academic-Lite Edition: Many hospital systems have caught on to the value of having interns and residents, including those staffing the ICU. They get paid very little, and even with the more modern work hour rules, they work almost non-stop. These programs are not typically affiliated with universities and may be in areas with a larger proportion of uninsured or under-insured patients. They do have to meet the accreditation requirements to run a residency but are often set up to offer practical training over academic training. The house staff here can be excellent and very dedicated (why else would they accept these conditions), but they are may not be the first-round draft picks either (why else would they accept these conditions).

ii. Private Hospitals

Private hospitals are owned by a corporation or organization. They manage what health insurance they accept and may not allow admission if you can't afford to be there. You may be imagining fountains in the lobby, curated art in the hallways, and a classical music quartet in the dining room. This may be true in a few high dollar famous hospitals, but all hospitals are typically extremely cost conscious. Since the reimbursement rate is determined by your diagnosis, they get paid the same with or without the quartet. If they have these perks, it is usually to entice more insured patients to have their elective surgeries with them rather than at their competitor a few blocks away. These perks exist because someone donated the money for these extras and got their name on a lobby or building (academic hospitals have also caught on to this facet of fund raising). This has little bearing on the actual care you get. Private hospitals may also be academic centers or affiliates of such centers.

> ***ICU Confidential Pay to Play Edition:*** Whether they take your insurance or not, every emergency department even in an out of network private hospital is obligated to provide emergency care and stabilize you if your situation is severe or life threatening, including for imminent childbirth. This is part of the **Emergency Medical Treatment and Labor Act** (**EMTALA**). They cannot turn you away, although they can and will try to collect on the bill. Once stabilized, they have the right to transfer you to a facility that takes your insurance (or if you are uninsured).

iii. Public Hospitals:

Public hospitals are owned and managed by the county or state government and are typically designated as community health trusts. They are sometimes referred to as county hospitals, and most are part of academic centers as they could not financially survive without house staff (residents, Interns, and medical students). These hospitals can be overwhelming, with older infrastructure, much more crowded conditions, and overworked staff. They can be large and specialized due to their sheer volume of patients and have scores of house staff to oversee the large number of patients who often have very advanced diseases and limited or no insurance. They often serve as a safety net for these patients (there goes the marble fountain budget).

Public hospitals also often have a private part either as a section or even a whole separate building with its own name. They tend to attract highly specialized physicians running research programs and working with new technologies, who take care of patients both in the public and private sections. As such, these types of public hospitals may offer the highest level of academic practice as well as procedures that may not be available at the stand-alone shiny hospital with spa services (think organ transplantation, advanced clinical research trials, and other resource intensive interventions).

> ***ICU Confidential County Edition:*** Public hospitals are generally great places to train as they provide a large number of patients who often have diseases that are very far along because of lack of prior access to healthcare. They are also tough places to train. Fortunately, they tend to attract supervising physicians that do what they do because they truly care about medicine, teaching, and taking care of patients as a calling. Not to say this isn't true for private practice or non-academic

center-based physicians; I've worked with many great docs on both sides. And, as noted, many physicians do go between both the public and private practice domains.

iv. Veteran's Administration (VA) Hospitals:

The VA hospital system is among the largest health networks in the country. Designed to serve the unique needs of patients who served in the U.S. armed forces, these hospitals offer the services found in any other hospital system in addition to specialized care for conditions more common in veterans. They span from small community hospitals to large **tertiary care** medical centers. Like all hospitals, quality varies according to each location. Some VA facilities are old, but some are modern masterpieces that rival the fanciest private hospitals.

The hospitals within the VA system share common organizational and policy structures. As a result, they have economies of scale. Many are part of academic teaching programs shared with the local university-based hospital. All in all, VA hospitals offer a tremendous set of resources and specialized care even if they may be harder to navigate. Active military members also have their own hospital systems.

v. Profit versus Not-for-Profit Hospitals:

The distinction between for-profit (private) and not-for-profit hospitals is more of a tax and legal one. All hospitals have to focus on their bottom lines. All hospitals have significant financial responsibilities and are constantly focused on efficiency. The main difference is that not-for-profit hospitals operate as non-profit corporations rather than being responsible to shareholders, and any positive income gets automatically re-invested in the community. By way of compensation, they receive significant tax exemptions and other benefits.

In contrast, for-profit systems function to make money for their owners and/or shareholders. They have to meet the same quality and safety standards, and they espouse similar goals of making your health their priority, of course. I will say, at least in my know-it-all opinion, the for-profit hospitals allow finances to drive their decisions in a much bigger way. It's as if they were there to...make a profit.

> ***ICU Confidential Best Places to Stay Edition:*** If you have a particularly specialized problem, you may be better off going to a brand name academic medical center. They may not be taking out an appendix every minute, but they have the world's experts in the disease you and only 9 other people have. The best place to be as a patient who needs advanced and complex care for "regular" problems is an academic medical center with a private hospital component where you are in the private hospital part. You get the best of both worlds with access to highly specialized care (the same doctors go between all parts of these centers), and a fancier lobby to boot.

F. E(lectronic)-ICU:

It was just a matter of time. In the era of systems efficiency and a shortage of ICU physicians, specialized remote monitoring systems have been developed where an intensivist physician oversees your care remotely. Yes, that's right, remotely, like tele-medicine on steroids. This typically involves a state-of-the-art control center with live remote feeds to the monitoring equipment in your room, including vital signs, a very high-definition camera, microphone, and more. The intensivist can talk to you, see you on video, and may even be able to connect to your television screen so you can see them.

The intensivist usually oversees dozens or more patients from different ICUs in different hospitals. Algorithms are built in to automatically alert the physician to a worrisome change in vital signs that can trigger a call to your nurse for further evaluation. Hands on adjustments in care, including procedures, are managed by the in-person physician, typically a hospitalist who is taking care of the rest of the hospital patients at the same time.

There are definite advantages to having this extra pair of eyes electronically looking over you when intensivists aren't available on site. This is especially true of rural hospitals that may have only a few ICU beds and can be a hundred miles from a larger center. The cost of an on-site intensivist can't be justified so e-ICU may fill the gap. There is of course a downside: imagine trying to have an end-of-life discussion with your TV. At least you can't be unplugged remotely...or can you?

G. Staffing Models

ICU staffing involves a lot of organization and can be dynamic depending on how many patients need care. As we'll soon discuss, ICUs are staffed by not only physicians, but also a variety of health professionals that specialize in the kind of care you need, like nurses, respiratory therapists, and pharmacists.

In general, ICU nurses work 12-hour shifts taking care of 2 patients, sometimes 3. If a patient is very medically active and requires ongoing assessments and interventions, they may get their own nurse (actually not a good sign). There is also a **Charge Nurse** overseeing the flow of activity throughout the ICU, who is ready to step in to help where needed.

Larger ICUs will also have their own **respiratory therapists**, or **RTs**, who help manage the ventilator and provide therapies to help your breathing. The RT also typically does 12-hour shifts. The number of other personnel, like pharmacists and physical therapists, can vary and these individuals may also be responsible for patients outside the ICU. The larger the ICU, the more likely these individuals will take care of ICU patients exclusively.

Physicians in academic centers have a physician and/or a physician-in-training physically in the hospital and assigned to the ICU 24/7. The physicians-in-training, or house staff, (interns and residents, see Chapter 4: Who's Who in the ICU) typically work 12-hour shifts, with a day team and night team. For larger places with multiple teams there is usually an early team and a late team during the day. The late team may do new patient admissions and urgent interventions until the night team arrives (often called **Night Float**). If **fellows** (post-residency subspecialty trainees) are part of the team, they are there for the day and may perform night coverage as well.

In places without house staff (interns, residents, fellows), an **attending** (senior) physician works in 12-hour shifts, typically doing several day (or night) shifts in a row so there is some continuity. The night intensivists may officially evaluate all their ICU patients (also called making **rounds**) but are more commonly there only for emergencies and to admit new patients. This is out of necessity, as night coverage may have one intensivist for every 2 or more present during the day. In some places where the volume of patients is lower, the intensivist is there during the day and on call from home during the night (this sucks for you and for them). In places with **Advanced Nurse Practitioners** (physician extenders, more on this in Chapter 4: Who's Who in the ICU), they usually mimic the schedules of house staff.

Subspecialists have their own coverage arrangements but are typically available 24/7 for consultations. Some busier specialty services stay at the facility overnight, and most are a phone call away. They typically see their hospital patients in the morning, before their clinics, or in the late afternoon. In an emergency, they come right away.

H. How the ICU Gets Paid

Nothing's free in this world (except true love and STIs). Next to the operating rooms, nothing's more expensive to run than the ICU. Aside from the physical plant, you need a whole slew of professionals who are typically on salary. The machines, the single-use items, the medications, all add up to big money. That's why your insurance is charged thousands of dollars per day just in rent. Add in charges for special procedures, medical devices, consultations, and more. In truth, however, the ICU rarely comes out financially ahead.

In the world of Medicare and the private insurers who take their lead from Medicare, your hospital gets a lump sum payment depending on your diagnosis. This is called a **diagnosis related group**, or **DRG** for short. There is an excessively complicated system of formulas and government regulations that control and determine who gets paid for what. For example, if you are admitted for dangerously low blood pressure (**shock**) from a kidney infection, the hospital gets a set amount of money whether you got so sick you ended up in the ICU on life support for a week, or you ended up in the ICU for a day because your blood pressure was a little soft (low). The hospital can get paid more when you are in the ICU, but you are definitely not there just to make the hospital money. You are there to survive and recover from your life-threatening illness, perhaps so you can come back and make them more money in the future.

I. Quality Markers

In the ICU, quality is defined in many ways. Being able to leave the hospital, and with good **functional status**, is on top of the list. How long you are on a ventilator, time in the ICU, and total time in the hospital, are also important quality markers. Whether you catch an infection from your catheter or ventilator (**hospital acquired infections**) counts too.

1. **Why the ICU saves lives:**
   This is hopefully self-evident. Closer, more specialized care delivered by individuals with significant expertise leads to better outcomes for patients that need it. Then the question is, why isn't every patient in the hospital an ICU patient from the moment they walk through the doors to the moment they go home. Certainly, cost and availability, but there's also another side...
2. **Why the ICU can be a dangerous place.**
   The most serious infections, constant interruptions to rest at all hours of the day and night, little to no privacy, being tied down by more wires and tubes than you can count – these are some of the consequences of all that extra care, and the source of expected complications from being in the ICU.

Quality is built into the framework of the following tenets:

i. Quality is Mortality

When someone is offered a lifesaving medication that needs careful monitoring and infusion through a special central IV line, or special life-support equipment like a ventilator or a special pump to support your heart function, the ICU is the place where these interventions are possible. Depending on the diagnosis that landed you there, your chance of survival without these interventions is significantly lower.

There are benchmarks for survival rates across different diagnoses, adjusted for how sick you are to begin with. These calculations take into account factors like your age, other medical problems (pre-existing conditions), and how bad you were functionally before you got to the ICU, among many other variables. All hospitals and their different services are measured against these benchmarks as their actual survival rates are compared to average or expected survival rates.

ii. Quality is How Long You Wait

When things need to get done quickly and comprehensively, the more staff you have and the better trained they are, the faster things can get done. For example, if you are showing signs of infection that can lead to sepsis, how quickly this is recognized and then how quickly it is treated can mean the difference between life and death. The same is true for treating heart attacks, strokes, and all sorts of potentially life-ending medical problems. While this starts in the ED when you arrive (see Chapter 2: Anatomy of a Hospital), the process continues upon admission to the hospital including the ICU. Testing is also prioritized for critical care patients, as are most interventions. ICU/VIP pass, coming through!

iii. Quality is Length of Stay

Like mortality rates, how long it takes you to get better when receiving specialized ICU care can be measured against an expected average while accounting for differences in medical history, age, and all sorts of factors. In high-quality ICUs, you can get better faster, and therefore to be discharged from the ICU after a shorter stay. (This presumes that you are not being discharged quickly because you suffered an avoidable death.).

iv. Quality is How Long You Are on a Ventilator

If you are on life support with a machine breathing for you, there are time- and data-proven factors that help liberate you from this interesting experience. Daily **sedation vacations** and **spontaneous breathing trials**, for example, can make a huge difference in coming off the ventilator sooner and with fewer complications (see Chapter 8: Life Support in the ICU). Duration on a ventilator given specific conditions is measured and compared to expected standards.

v. Quality is the Prevention of Complications

Every intervention in the ICU has potential complications. From infections that occur from large catheters in your blood vessels (**central lines**), to skin breakdown from pressure sores, to ventilator related infections, avoiding or, at least, minimizing these complications is a quality maker.

vi. Quality is a Multi-disciplinary Approach

A team approach to your care carries enormous benefits. On the medical side, each individual brings with them their experience and expertise. When medical issues are discussed in a collaborative way, better outcomes ensue. Likewise, input from the specialist pharmacist, the physical therapist, the respiratory therapist, and other professional staff enhances and individualizes your treatment plan. Good leadership ensures that the team doesn't get stuck in the analysis paralysis zone or the just-do-it impulsive zone.

vii. Quality is Staffing

Having the right expertise from nursing to pharmacists to intensivists makes all the difference. How many patients each staff member is caring for is just as important. What's the use of having an expert if they are spread way too thin to make a difference in your care?

There are quality guidelines for patient-to-intensive care physician ratios, as well as nurse-to-patient ratios. The Society of Critical Care Medicine® and the LeapFrog Group® are two organizations that use data driven quality markers to determine what makes a difference in your chance of survival.

> ***ICU Confidential Less is More Edition:*** The best outcomes in general are with *a closed ICU in an academic center staffed by on-site board-certified intensivists with a 14-patient limit per intensivist.* Some larger hospitals have an intensivist covering all their ICUs in general (think 50-60 or more patients). They are just there for emergencies, and while this is better than not having them, it's not the same as having a closed ICU system.

viii. Quality is All of the Above

Quality Indicators are monitored by the hospital's **Quality Assurance** department. All unexpected medical complications are also reported to the state, and the federal government also compiles quality indicators and reports them at:

https://www.medicare.gov/care-compare/resources/hospital/overall-star-rating.

On a broader and less specific scale, many of the national rankings (think US News & World Report®, Leapfrog®, Healthgrades®, Newsweek® and the like) use these and other indicators and tell you who is in the top whatever percent for one specialty or another. These organizations rank hospitals using Medicare claims, other quality metrics, and patient data that may or may not directly apply to your ICU stay. Perhaps like college or automobile rankings, the information may certainly have value but should be looked at in the context of your individual medical situation.

ICU Confidential Yelp Me Edition: Of course, there's also the local reputation of your hospital. You probably have some idea of which place is better than another. Ask the insiders – physicians and especially nurses will know which hospital they would or wouldn't go to as patients. As much as I hate to say it given how much I worship at the data throne, there's usually a reason for that.

ICU Confidential Not My Job Edition: While how good your food tastes, how soft your blanket is, whether you get HGTV® on your hospital TV (why do so few people *List It*?) may be your primary quality markers, your ICU physicians usually don't care about this as we try to save your life. While most of us are pretty nice about it, please save those concerns for your nurse, your tech, or your blog. Please also include the fact that you are alive to complain about it, and who got you there. *Meeeow!*

4 Who's Who in the ICU

The ICU is a complex environment with lots of moving parts. To make all of them work, you need a team of professionals all working together so you or your loved one can get better and leave! Below you'll find a description of who these individuals are, and what they do.

A. Nurses and Nursing Assistants

Nurses are an amazing group of people. They dedicate their professional lives to caring for their patients through thick and thin, often putting their patients' wellbeing before their own (remember the COVID-19 pandemic?). They provide comfort, they save lives, they advocate for their patients, and yes, they even maintain your hygiene. ICU nurses are an elite group within the nursing family.

To be an ICU nurse requires special training and experience. ICU nurses with **critical care certification** (**CCRN**) must meet a minimum of 1750 hours providing care at the bedside of people who are deemed critically ill. They have to have a minimum of 5 years of practical experience, and they must pass an intensive exam. After obtaining their certification, these CCRNs must maintain it with a continued set of requirements. Not all ICUs are able to be staffed by CCRNs, but this designation is certainly a mark of advanced experience and expertise.

Many nurses also have additional competence for certain interventions. For example, nurses in the cardiothoracic ICU would have special expertise with machines and medications for patients on advanced heart therapies. ICU nurses may also specialize in other complex treatments, like **dialysis** or chemotherapy infusions.

ICUs also have nurse's assistants. While they do not administer medication, they can help with feeding and cleaning duties, as well as taking blood sugar readings, and with getting various things that you may need (like a new remote control for your TV or just a little extra conversation).

More than anyone else on the team, your nurse will spend more time at your bedside. Everything they do can be put into one of three main categories: assess and report on your condition, provide comfort and care, and carry out the physician's orders. ICU nurses have many responsibilities. This is by no means an exhaustive list, but they include:

1. Assess and report:
    - ♥ Talk to you and actually listen
    - ♥ Monitor vital signs
    - ♥ Assess neurologic, cardiac, respiratory, and every other aspect specific to why you are in the ICU
    - ♥ Communicate with your family
    - ♥ Call for help when needed
2. Comfort and therapy:
    - ♥ Help explain what's going on
    - ♥ Help with pain
    - ♥ Help you move
    - ♥ Help you eat
    - ♥ Help with your bathroom needs
    - ♥ Help you stay clean
3. Carry out physician's orders
    - ♥ Give medications and assess response
    - ♥ Accompany you to testing and procedures
    - ♥ Help your doctors for bedside exams and procedures
    - ♥ Keep track of consultants and other professionals
    - ♥ Question/confirm orders that don't seem quite right

As physicians, we rely on nurses to make sure our patients are safe and getting what they need, and to let us know if your condition is changing in real time, not just when we are directly seeing you. Nurses participate in rounds, in family meetings, and in procedures. In a well-run ICU, nurses are an absolutely essential core part of the team and are treated as such.

ICU Nursing Confidential: Your nurses are your main points of contact in an ICU. They usually take care of you and only one other patient for 12 hours and will inherit you on their next shift the next day. Be kind to them and they will be kind to you, but if you do have friction, be honest with them and discuss your concerns. If you are not satisfied, insist on speaking with the nurse supervisor. If all else fails, insist on speaking to the nursing manager. Since your nurse does not administratively answer to or work for your physician, we often go up the nursing chain of command just as you would. If you are not getting satisfaction for a major concern, however, your attending physician has to step in.

ICU Confidential The Nurses Know Edition: If you really want to know who the good doctors are in your hospital, ask an experienced nurse. They work with us hand in hand and can tell pretty quickly if we know what we're doing, if we let our ego get in the way, and if we're there for the right reasons. There is no better compliment a physician will get than to be recommended by an ICU nurse.

B. Therapists

The term **therapist** applies to a category of professionals who administer the many therapies available in an ICU, from providing breathing treatments to helping with mobility. While they cannot order medications or procedures, they help get you to your health goals in a variety of essential ways and are an integral part of your recovery. This is not to be confused with mental health therapists, such as psychologists and counselors. Those are discussed separately in Chapter 5: Other Physicians You May Encounter in the ICU.

i. Respiratory Therapists

As a pulmonologist (lung doc), respiratory therapists (**RTs**) play a special role in my patients' care, and nowhere is this more essential than in the ICU. For patients who are not on a ventilator, RTs provide **nebulized** medications (medications that you breathe in) and oxygen therapy in its many forms. They also set up and troubleshoot therapies like **high flow oxygen** and **non-invasive ventilation** (like **BPAP**, discussed in Appendix I: Machines and Things). They help suction your airways to clear out phlegm, offer **chest physiotherapy,** and obtain **blood gases**.

If you are sick enough to need life support, RTs also assist in **intubations** and set up the **ventilator** as this is such a specialized type of equipment that running it needs its own training. In some hospitals, RTs also perform **intubations**. As physicians, we rely on their expertise to troubleshoot and adjust the ventilator settings, as well as to adjust ventilator breathing tubes (**endotracheal tubes**). RTs also help us figure out when you are ready to come off the ventilator. More information on all this in Appendix I: Machines and Things.

ii. Physical Therapists and Occupational Therapists

Physical therapy is an essential part of your medical care, including in the ICU. Physical therapists diagnose and treat people who have injuries and other health-related conditions that limit their ability to physically function. In the ICU, physical therapy often centers on getting very sick people moving again. This can be as simple as exercises in bed to walking the hallway (often with lots of IV poles in tow). Sometimes, just sitting at the edge of the bed can be a huge accomplishment.

These therapies are not just essential for stroke or trauma patients. It's been consistently shown that the sooner you can get a patient physically moving, the better they do, no matter the underlying diagnosis. Of course, you have to be safe enough to do this. This includes meeting criteria like being off high dose **pressors**, having reasonable oxygen levels, and having a reasonable mental status. While there are rare situations where people can participate in physical therapy out of their beds while on **ventilators** (or even **ECMO**), these are very specific situations where patients are typically on long-term support but are awake and otherwise stable enough to undergo therapy.

Occupational therapy focuses on helping people do the simple but essential physical things they need to do in their daily lives. In the ICU, occupational therapists often work with patients on everyday activities like manipulating utensils or getting dressed. While physical therapists focus on movement, occupational therapists focus on daily function. A patient usually has both physical and occupational therapy needs and so they are often ordered together.

> ***ICU Confidential Get Off the Couch Edition:*** Your physician and nurse may stress the importance of getting out of bed even just to a recliner. I can't stress how important this can be in your recovery. You may have pain — we'll control it. You may be weak — we'll help with movement. You may be depressed — moving can actually help. Whatever the barrier, being laid up even for a couple of days results in muscle wasting and impairs overall fitness. When the physical and occupational therapists come around, please do your best to participate and let them help you (literally) get on your feet. Please do wait for help and don't try it yourself — you're guaranteed to trip on one of the many tubes you're connected to. Remember, the more enthusiastic you are in your recovery, the more enthusiastic we are in your recovery.

iii. Speech Therapists

In the ICU, speech therapists (aka **speech-language pathologists**) are often called upon to assess your ability to speak and swallow, performing what we refer to as a **swallow evaluation.** Swallowing is a complex activity requiring coordination of many muscles. While evaluating your ability to swallow is essential with stroke and other neurologic conditions, it's also really important after you've been on a ventilator, as your throat and vocal cords can be affected by the endotracheal tube.

To be ready to pass a swallow evaluation, you also have to be awake and not overly confused, and generally stable enough in other ways like blood pressure and oxygen levels. Sometimes a more invasive evaluation is needed using a fiberoptic scope that can visualize the vocal cords as you swallow (called a **fiberoptic endoscopic evaluation of swallowing** or **FEES** [more in Appendix II: Common Procedures in the ICU]).

In the special circumstance of a tracheostomy tube, the speech therapist assists with a **speech valve** (a **Passy-Muir Valve**) and helps train patients to talk through the tracheostomy. In patients using their natural airway, speech therapists also help with speech/voice issues.

iv. Other Therapists

Some hospitals have music therapists, art therapists, dog therapy, volunteers and more. They all bring an extra dimension to helping our patients with their cognitive and emotional stress. Some institutions are lucky enough to have them and they can contribute greatly to the mental well-being of patients and staff, including in the ICU.

C. Pharmacists

Medications have become more and more complex, and when you get into the ICU, it's on a whole other level (see Appendix III: Medication in the ICU). There are a slew of intravenous medications to be monitored and constantly adjusted, the interactions to be kept track of, and the blood levels to be checked.

ICU pharmacists play an essential role in all the above. Like nurses, they are typically part of the daily rounds with the ICU team and offer truly important input into the hour-by-hour care of the patient. In most hospitals, they are also responsible for calculating and mixing IV feeding (**total parenteral nutrition** or **peripheral parenteral nutrition**; see Appendix II: Common Procedures in the ICU for more information).

D. Dieticians or Nutritionists

Dieticians advise your medical team on how many and what kind of calories you will need. If you are being fed through a nasal or oral tube that goes into your stomach (I'm sorry), a dietician will help manage the type and amount of formula. If you need nutritional support through the IV, they work with your pharmacist to create the best formulation. If you are awake and eating, they also advise you about special diets for diabetes, kidney disease, heart disease, and other conditions.

> ***ICU Confidential Unhappy Meal Edition:*** Few things make your health care providers cringe quite like seeing fast food wrappers in your room, especially if you're there for a heart attack, stroke, or diabetic crisis. Sometimes, it's a matter of education, but most times you know better; it's kind of like showing up to my lung clinic and smoking a cigarette in the waiting room. We do judge. Ironically, fast food (donuts, muffins, etc.), are perfectly acceptable to bring for the staff.

E. Social Workers and Case Managers

When we think of social workers, we often imagine an individual coming in to check on a person's safety in their home environment, helping someone through a difficult time in their lives, or helping people navigate the world of social safety net programs. In the ICU, everything is taken to the next level.

First and foremost, social workers do provide emotional and psychological support and care for patients and their families. In the ICU, this gets intense! Some hospitals have a **licensed clinical social worker (LCSW)** assigned to every ICU patient. They require a master's or doctoral degree in social work and have a long list of qualifications to do what they do. They help families deal with impending loss, serve an important role in goals of care discussions, and help locate and organize things like living wills. They identify health care proxies (see Chapter 10: Code Status Definitions and Difficult Decisions) and serve as an information bridge for families and patients. They will typically meet every patient coming into the ICU and identify what specific things they can help with.

While the social worker focuses on psychosocial support for patients and families, a **case manager** typically coordinates the medical aspects of your situation. The case manager works on insurance coverage to help you figure out how to pay for your care (and to help the hospital get payment). Many treatments require specific insurance approvals (think organ transplant but also think about specialized medications that will have to be continued after you leave the ICU), and your insurance determines if this treatment will be covered. If you don't have insurance, the case manager works to qualify you for the appropriate safety net program. In some institutions, the social worker and the case manager are the same individual.

Another essential part of what social workers and case managers do is prepare you for discharge. They have the essential role of making sure you and your family have all the resources you need to safely transition to home, a rehabilitation hospital, **long term acute care hospital**, nursing home, or **hospice**. They help families coordinate the social aspects of their medical conditions and to navigate the insurance resources to see which places and services are covered, and what your family may need once you leave the ICU.

F. Physicians and Advanced Practice Providers

Care in the ICU is driven by many individuals in many disciplines, all working together to get you through your medical crisis. The discipline that oversees this care, that drives, coordinates, and decides on the tests and the therapies, and that is ultimately responsible for the medical or surgical decisions, is the physician team.

In smaller ICUs, this is a simple team of one main physician (the **attending**) working with your nurse and pharmacist. Many larger ICUs in non-academic/non-university-based systems also rely on physician extenders or **advanced practice providers**, such as **nurse practitioners**, **physician assistants,** or **advanced practice registered nurses**.

Academic institutions typically have a whole team of physicians (and medical students) at various stages of their training all under the ultimate supervision of the attending physician. Depending on the institution, they have more or less autonomy (both approaches have their advantages and disadvantages).

i. Medical Students, Interns, Residents, and Fellows

In a typical academic ICU, there is a hierarchy designed to meet the needs of patient care while offering individuals at different levels of training the opportunity to learn. Usually, the lower the level of training, the more time that individual has with you as you will be among the only patients they are responsible for. The higher the level of training, the more patients that individual has; they will typically play a more supervisory role.

Interns, residents, and fellows are collectively known as **house staff.**

a. Medical Students

Medical students assigned to you are going through their 4 year medical school training, and you are meeting them in their 3rd or 4th year in their clinical or hands-on rotations. A medical student will often only be following a couple of patients at a time. As a patient, you will get most of their undivided attention while they learn about your childhood illnesses, your hobbies, your daily routines, and your life story. In complex medical mysteries, it sometimes takes that level of granularity to figure out what's wrong (usually not, though). The medical student can be the essential information gatherer. While they do not make any medical decisions or have any ability to enter orders, medical students do have the ability (and responsibility) to get more help quickly when you need it.

b. Interns

The intern has graduated medical school and is still getting used to being called "doctor." Interns are also the main information gatherers, and they have the responsibility of entering the orders, making the phone calls, arranging for tests, and making sure all those check marks are marked off the to-do list. As they get further along in the academic year, they formulate treatment plans and become more proactive.

c. Residents

The resident takes on a more supervisory role. In the medical ICU, they are in their 2nd or 3rd year of their 3-year training in internal medicine. The medical ICU is a large part of their training, but like when they were medical students, they also rotate through the general hospital wards, outpatient clinics, and a slew of subspecialty rotations.

In a surgical ICU, these are individuals in general or specialty surgical training programs or in an anesthesia training program who are going through their ICU rotations. Residents are also honing their procedure skills, including helping interns with large IV lines (**central lines**), **arterial lines**, and with inserting needles and catheters wherever else they are needed (see Appendix I: Machines and Things).

The residents supervise the interns and medical students and help lay out the medical thought processes and drive medical decisions for your care. Along with the medical student and intern, they are typically your primary point of day-to-day medical contact.

d. Fellows

A fellowship is the subspecialty training individuals get once they've finished their residency in general medical training. For example, a qualified internist after 3 years of internal medicine training can chose to do several years of further subspecialty training to become a cardiologist, gastroenterologist, or a critical care specialist (intensivist).

For ICUs in larger training institutions, you will have a critical care fellow overseeing the team. This will be an internal medicine physician now in specialty training in the medical ICU, or an anesthesiologist in the surgical ICU. The fellow is a supervisor making sure the residents and interns (and medical students) are all doing what they are supposed to, including supervising the procedures or performing them themselves if they are complicated or higher level.

They also oversee the most pivotal conversations and make sure you are fully informed of your medical situation. If the medical students and interns are privates first class, and the senior resident is the sergeant, then the fellow is a lieutenant.

Outside of formal rounds where the whole team is conferencing on each patient, the fellow is typically the right-hand person to the attending physician (whom we will meet shortly) and serves to update them directly.

ii. Advanced Practice Providers – Nurse Practitioners, Physician Assistants, and Advanced Practice Registered Nurses

Advanced practice providers (**APPs**) work directly with the attending so that together they can manage a greater number of patients in the ICU. APPs are an extra pair of skilled hands that help address physician shortages, allow for more time and attention to the individual patients, and contribute to improved outcomes, especially in hospitals without house staff.

APPs include nurse practitioners (**NPs**), physician assistants (**PAs**), and advanced practice registered nurses, (**APRNs**). APRNs have a registered nurse (**RN**) license, clinical experience, and a master's degree in nursing. (There are also different types of APRNS who provide care outside the ICU including certified nurse practitioners, certified nurse midwifes, and nurse anesthetists).

NPs and PAs have similar education and training requirements, including taking on specialized training and experience in the ICU setting. Most APPs in the ICU are also certified to perform procedures including central and arterial lines, and they get really good at them.

Many hospitals employ APPs to help manage their ICUs. They can work as part of an academic team, or in parallel with them, taking care of their own set of patients. For the purposes of an ICU, APPs essentially function as the combined intern-resident-fellow for your care.

As well trained as these professionals may be, it is important to understand that APPs did not go to medical school and are not typically licensed to practice independently in the ICU setting. This is not to take away from their importance; they can be absolutely essential to your care and can be very experienced and dedicated. But they are not physicians.

iii. Attending Physician

The attending physician is the person ultimately responsible for your care. While they work as part of the team that is taking care of you, it's their name (and license) that is at the top on your chart and they are ultimately responsible for your care. They are the captain of the medical team ship, overseeing the functions of all the other team members.

When an attending physician has completed their critical care fellowship specialty training they are known as an **intensivist**. Most medical intensivists do combined training for pulmonary (lung) medicine as well (3 years instead of 2) after completing their internal medicine training. Most surgical intensivists go the anesthesia or general surgery training route.

Larger academic and private hospitals will have an intensivist as the attending physician in charge of the ICU. Some places where this is not available staff the ICU with a general practice physician or are "open," meaning that the hospitalist or primary care physician or surgeon of the patient is the same in ICU as in the general wards. In this scenario, these ICUs typically rely on individual consultants to help guide care (see the open or closed ICU discussion in Chapter 3: What is an ICU and Why am I There). Some open ICUs have intensivists as consultants where they co-manage the patients but where the general physician has the ultimate say.

The attending physician ultimately guides your medical decisions by supervising the entirety of the ICU team on formal rounds and beyond. They often supervise or perform the higher complexity procedures (like **intubations**), participate in the most serious aspects of discussions of your care, offer formal teaching to the team, and oversee the big picture decisions. They are also there to make certain that no aspect of your care is overlooked, like making sure you are on the most appropriate medications, are getting the right therapists on board, and even that you are having regular bowel movements (yes, I do ask this of every patient during rounds).

Depending on the institution and the individual, attendings can be hands-on to different degrees. They can oversee a larger number of patients and offer the benefit of their expertise because of the hierarchy described above. It's important to recognize that face-to-face time with your attending is only a small proportion of their role in your care.

As attending physicians, we can't fix the cafeteria food or prevent the blood draw technician from waking you at 5 am, but we are there to make sure all the members of the medical team work to get you successfully through the ICU experience.

ICU Confidential Consulting Edition: Subspecialty or consulting services such as cardiology, gastroenterology, and so forth have a similar structure to that described above in larger institutions. In smaller hospitals, sometimes you only get the attending subspecialty physician, possibly along with an advanced practice provider. In either scenario, the attending is ultimately responsible for making the final recommendations. In some institutions, the fellow essentially runs the service, and the attending gets more directly involved only if there's a problem. When a fellow or APP makes a recommendation, you can absolutely ask to speak directly with the attending physician especially if you have reservations about your care.

ICU Confidential Who Supervises the Supervisor: There is typically a critical care physician who is the director of the ICU. Aside from taking their turn as an attending, they are also responsible for policies and procedures, quality, patient safety, and staff conflict resolution. Above them is the chair of the department. In different organizations, this is the Chief of Pulmonary or of Subspecialties or of Surgery. Then there's who all the physicians ultimately report to, the Chief of Staff, who may then report to the hospital president or CEO. If you do have an issue with the attending physician, the person you should speak to first is none of those (as they will have no idea of your specific care and may default to a defensive posture); it's actually the **ombudsman**. More on this in Chapter 12: Advice for Getting the Best Experience.

G. And Finally...

I would be remiss if I didn't highlight all the professionals usually working behind the scenes to make the hospital run so that it can maintain an ICU. The myriads of engineers, IT professionals, security staff, cooks and servers, administrative professionals, environmental workers, operators and many technicians that are needed to ensure that you get the care you need will make your head spin (and maybe justify your bill?). This also includes safety and quality officers (usually physicians and specially trained administrators), lawyers, coders and insurance professionals, and many more. While you won't see most of these individuals directly, our job as medical professionals would not be possible without them.

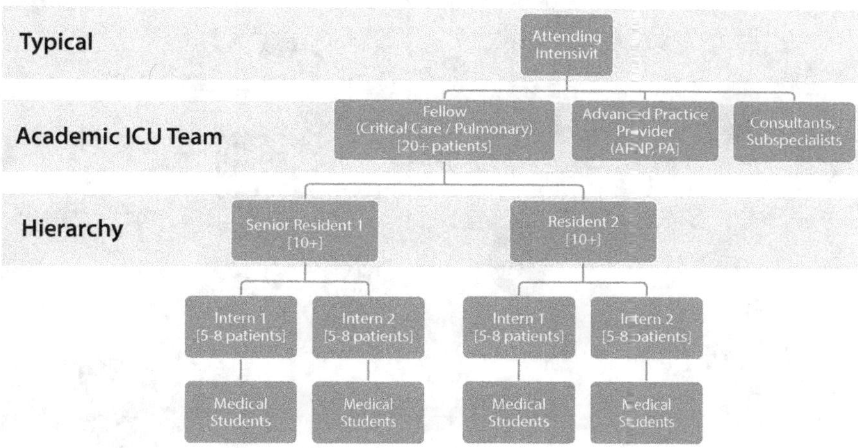

Training Day(cades)

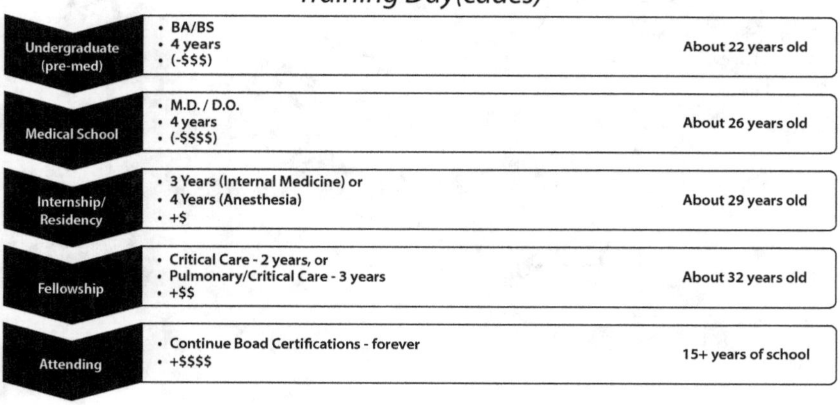

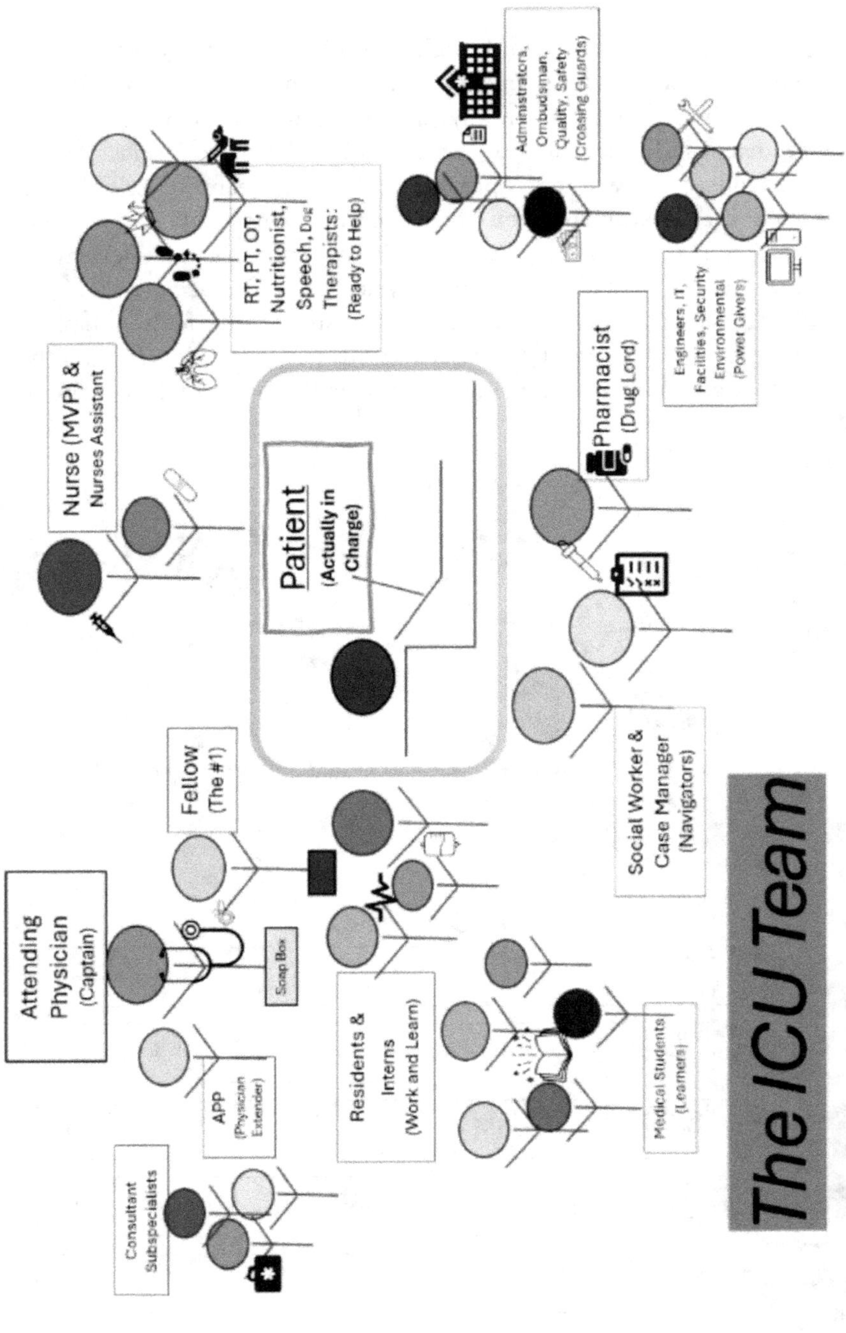
The ICU Team
Attending Physician (Captain)
Soap Box
Fellow (The #1)
APP (Physician Extender)
Consultant Subspecialists
Residents & Interns (Work and Learn)
Medical Students (Learners)
Patient (Actually in Charge)
Nurse (MVP) & Nurses Assistant
RT, PT, OT, Nutritionist, Speech, Dog Therapists: (Ready to Help)
Social Worker & Case Manager (Navigators)
Pharmacist (Drug Lord)
Administrators, Ombudsman, Quality, Safety (Crossing Guards)
Engineers, IT, Facilities, Security Environmental (Power Givers)

5 Other Physicians You May Encounter in the ICU

As we've outlined in the Who's Who in the ICU (Chapter 4), there is a cadre of providers caring for you in the ICU. These subspecialists are called consultants and will be added to your care team when called in by your main physician. Below is a list of the types of physicians (in alphabetical order) and a brief description of what they do. This will help orient you to the different teams of doctors you may encounter (or sometimes need to ask for).

Anesthesiologists

Anesthesiologists help put you to sleep during surgery and other procedures. In the SICU, the intensivist is usually an anesthesiologist who works hand in hand with the surgeon. As the airway experts, anesthesiologists are also there to help when you need to be **intubated** and placed on a **ventilator** and come help when someone else (pulmonologist or emergency department physician) is having trouble. They can also specialize in pain management and provide nerve blocks and other procedures including in the ICU.

Cardiologists

These heart specialists are usually the primary drivers of your ICU interventions if you are there for a heart attack, heart failure, or arrhythmia. If you happen to develop one of these issues while in the ICU for other reasons, the cardiologists are there to help as well. They come in several types according to their skill set. We call interventional cardiologists to open coronary arteries and fix heart valves with catheters (plumbers), electrophysiologists to fix your arrhythmia with shock or ablation (electricians), heart failure specialists to manage advanced heart therapies (mechanics), and even pre-transplant specialists when replacement may be needed (warranty department). Larger institutions have separate sub-sub-specialists for all your cardiology needs, each with a tag-along team of house staff and medical students.

Emergency Department Physicians

While staffing the emergency department, some facilities depend on emergency department (**ED**) physicians to intubate patients on the hospital ward or ICU in an emergency. They may be part of the **code blue** team that responds to medical emergencies on the hospital wards, and, in smaller hospitals, this often includes the ICU after hours when an intensive care physician isn't physically present.

Gastroenterologists

These are the digestive system specialists, treating medical problems from your esophagus down to your rectum, along with all the different organs that participate in processing what you eat (like the pancreas, liver, and gallbladder). In the ICU they are typically there to help manage gastrointestinal (**GI**) bleeding, liver failure, gallbladder disease, and all sorts of issues dealing with your gut. Gastroenterologists help determine if an **endoscopy** (camera down your throat and into your stomach) or **colonoscopy** (camera up your bottom and into your colon) is indicated and are the ones who perform it. If your GI problem requires surgery, the appropriate surgical specialist becomes involved.

Hematologists/Oncologists

Hematology physicians deal with all sorts of disorders of the blood, including certain blood-related cancers like **leukemia** and **lymphoma**. Hematologists are also called in for low blood counts (such as **anemia**) and high blood counts (such as **polycythemia**).

Oncologists deal with solid organ tumors, their treatment, and related complications. They may even start or continue chemotherapy while you are in the ICU. They are also invaluable in helping establish prognosis and assisting families in recognizing when palliation is the best option.

A **radiation oncologist** may also become involved in your care if radiation therapy is recommended for your cancer. Although technically a radiology specialist, they may become an essential part of your cancer treatment team.

Infectious Disease Physicians

Your intensivist or hospitalist physician is capable of treating infections with guideline driven antibiotic choices. But, when the antibiotics management gets complicated, the infectious disease (**ID**) physician gets consulted. This has definitely been the case during pandemics (think MERS, H1N1, certainly COVID-19). If you are a transplant patient or on chemotherapy with significant immune deficiencies, the ID physician also gets involved. Some very heavy duty or specialized antibiotics require direct approval from the ID consultant so as to ensure proper use of these more complex medications.

Interventional Radiologists

These are radiologists that have advanced training in using imaging for biopsies and other interventions. Using tools like ultrasound and CT guidance, these physicians are able to offer minimally invasive biopsies, catheter insertions, and even taking out clots from blood vessels. Interventional radiology (**IR**) has blossomed as a field and has replaced many surgeries.

Nephrologists

If your kidneys are failing, your ICU team will do an evaluation that may include an ultrasound, along with urine and blood tests. Sometimes it's obvious why the kidneys are failing, and your ICU physicians intervene to turn the situation around. If it gets complicated, a kidney specialist or nephrologist is called in.

If you are on or need to start **dialysis**, a nephrologist will absolutely get involved. The ICU team usually sets up the access (dialysis) catheter, and the nephrologist guides the details of dialysis. There is usually a dialysis nurse that's part of their team to set up the dialysis machine. For continuous dialysis, the specially trained ICU nurse usually manages the dialysis machine.

Neurologists

These are brain and nervous system specialists. Their help is invaluable in managing events like acute strokes, brain bleeds, and seizures, often working in conjunction with neuro-interventional radiologists and neurosurgeons. In most facilities, they are also the experts in obtaining spinal fluid samples performing a special procedure called a **lumbar puncture**. Neurologists are also experts in interpreting the squiggly lines collecting brain function data from those wires glued to your scalp (**electroencephalogram** or **EEG**), usually looking for seizures. They are also often called upon to help discern why you are confused (due to medications, primary brain disease, or **toxic encephalopathy**, general code name for 'confused because you're sick'). Neurologists are also the experts in confirming **brain death**.

Psychiatrists and Psychologists

In the ICU, psychiatrists often help in managing acute psychotic episodes, as well as in helping patients after a suicide attempt. They also play an important role in determining a patient's capacity to make their own medical decisions. While a psychiatrist's approval is not required to involuntarily commit you because you are a danger to yourself or others (which prevents you from leaving the hospital for up to 72 hours, depending on the state), psychiatrists can help when the primary hospital physician isn't completely sure.

Psychiatrists also help manage severe complications from psychiatric medications, like unintended overdose and drug reactions including **serotonin syndrome** and **neuroleptic malignant syndrome**. Finally, psychiatrists can help deal with the high grade anxiety and depression that is unfortunately common in the ICU, especially during prolonged stays.

Psychologists also play an essential role in any ICU lucky enough to have them. While they are not medical doctors (they are PhD or PsyD doctors), they have specific training in providing mental health support to patients and families, addressing issues like anxiety and depression through counseling and psychotherapy.

Pulmonologists

Always the coolest doctors in the hospital, we are your lung specialists. As you already read, your MICU intensivist typically has a dual specialty that includes pulmonary medicine. This is for historical and practical reasons (ICU care often involves treating severe breathing problems and using the **ventilator**). In the SICU, the intensivist typically has an anesthesia dual specialty, so they definitely know their way around the ventilator – you don't need a separate pulmonologist for this.

If you have other lung issues like advanced **COPD** or **emphysema**, difficult to control **asthma**, a spot in the lungs that needs a biopsy, or if a second opinion is needed for why you aren't able to wean from the ventilator, a pulmonologist may be called in if not already on your case. If you need a scope inserted into your airways for inspection or a good cleanout, the MICU or SICU intensivist usually does this as well.

If it's a more complicated situation where a biopsy or other airway intervention is required, a pulmonologist with extra bronchoscopy training is your specialist of choice. Higher specialty centers have **interventional pulmonologists** that have extra training in fancier bronchoscopy interventions like airway stents and lasers. These procedures are usually elective and are performed on patients not admitted to the hospital, but sometimes may be required acutely in the ICU.

Rheumatologists

Physicians that deal with the immune system when it goes haywire and starts attacking your own organs and tissues are rheumatologists. While there are rheumatologic emergencies like acute inflammation of the arteries (**arteritis**) or kidneys (**scleroderma** renal crisis), rheumatologists also help manage your chronic immune disorders that still need care while you're in the ICU.

Surgeons

If you are in the surgical ICU (SICU) it's because a surgeon has operated on you or will be operating on you very shortly. There are many types of surgeons, each specializing in different body areas and techniques. A cardiothoracic surgeon may operate on your heart and lungs, an orthopedic surgeon on bones, a neurosurgeon on the brain and nerves, and so on. Some will practice in a special type of surgical ICU (like the cardiothoracic ICU for heart surgery patients).

In the medical ICU (MICU), surgeons often fulfill essential roles in your care as well. Surgical issues come up when you are being treated for medical problems, and a surgical intervention becomes lifesaving (think bowel strangulation requiring a **colectomy**, or **appendicitis** requiring an **appendectomy**). If so, you go to the operating room (OR) and come back to the SICU. Surgeons also participate in other important ways to consult on problems so they don't become surgical, like wound care (plastic surgery, general surgery), evaluation for blood vessel problems (vascular surgery), damage to hands (hand surgeons), or when you need to proceed to a tracheostomy (ENT surgeons usually do this, although some intensivists also have this training).

Wound Care Specialists

Wound care physicians and nurses are specialty providers with training and experience for complex wounds. They manage the choice and application of different medications, dressings and materials matched to your wound and give specific instructions for the ICU team to follow. They can recommend different **wound vacuums** and specialty mattresses as well.

Sometimes wounds need to be surgically cleaned out (**debrided**) or require other surgical interventions. Depending on where the wound is and what hospital you're in, a wound specialist, or a general or plastic surgeon may be called in to intervene.

> ***ICU Confidential Pain in the Butt Edition:*** Pressure wounds, or bedsores, on your lower back (**sacral ulcers**) and **heel ulcers** are not uncommon in patients with prolonged periods of limited mobility, as during a critical illness. Chronic malnutrition, difficulty maintaining hygiene, and failure to thrive add to the risk. Chronically ill patients cared for at home or in nursing homes can develop pressure wounds over weeks and months. They can be a source of infection that leads to sepsis, which lands or keeps you in the ICU. This can be prevented by vigilance, body position adjustments and turning every 2 hours, special mattresses, and other interventions. The development of pressure wounds is considered a quality marker and these types of complications, while common, can be prevented or at least markedly reduced with the measures noted above. It's important to document the presence or absence of pressure wounds on admission or transfer

to the hospital; ICUs usually document and photograph these on every admission (it wasn't us!).

Other Specialists

Almost any subspecialist may have a need to practice in the ICU. From the ophthalmologist to the podiatrist, when the situation calls for it, the subspecialist is asked to consult and offer their specialized advice. After all, if you're fighting off **sepsis,** you could still have still have a corneal abrasion or an infected toenail.

ICU Confidential Limited Edition: Keep in mind that not all facilities have access to all possible subspecialists, and those that do may have limited interventions. This is part of why certain facilities have designations like Stroke Center or Transplant Center. If you require services or specialists that are not available where you are currently at, and these services make the difference between recovery and not, you or your physician may request a hospital-to-hospital transfer.

ICU Confidential Who You Gonna Call Edition: The threshold for calling in a consultant varies by provider and institution. Some intensivist physicians call a specialist when they need a procedure only the specialist can perform. Others "pan-consult" and have a specialist on every organ just in case (more typical in private practice and open ICU systems). Most are somewhere in the middle, calling the specialist when the first- or second-line therapies aren't working and hopefully before a procedure is needed. If you are in a situation where you really do want that extra layer of expertise, don't be shy. Just politely ask your main doctor in the ICU to call in a specialist and your intensivist or general hospital physician is more than likely to oblige.

6 What To Expect Throughout the Day

Don't panic - it's going to be okay. Whether your first experience in the ICU is when you initially regain consciousness, or you were aware of your transport from the ED, recovery room, or hospital ward, it's good to get oriented in your new space and familiarize yourself with the ICU routines.

A. Arriving in a Strange Place

If you are conscious on arrival to the ICU, you will see that your transporter will be met by a group of people in your room that will transition you from whatever bed you came in and start hooking up the many sensors that come with your ICU stay. These are the nurses and nurses' aides that come together to get you set up.

They will glue sensors to your chest for heart monitoring (continuous **EKG** or **electrocardiogram**), place a probe on your finger or earlobe to measure oxygen saturation and pulse (**pulse oximeter**), and switch your oxygen cannula or mask to the supply built into the wall. Your calves will likely be wrapped in an inflatable material held together by Velcro® that will squeeze them periodically to prevent blood clots (**sequential compression stockings**). A blood pressure cuff completes the ensemble. Any drains and other catheters will also be switched over.

You will probably notice that your ICU hospital bed is larger, has railings that prevent you from falling (and from escaping), and has a number of buttons to control the position of the head and legs. A call button with a nursing symbol is usually built into the bed railing as well. The call button is also available on a wired remote control that accesses the lights and television functions.

The hallway wall will likely be an all-glass sliding door with minimal privacy. Above you and to your side, a monitor will hang from the ceiling displaying your vital signs with wires attached to the above-mentioned sensors. A number of **IV (intravenous)** poles housing medication pumps will flank your bed. Bags and bottles of medications and IV fluids may be hanging from those poles with tubing connecting to your IV catheter(s). Both the monitor and the IV poles will be making some beeping noises, to keep you company. The room will also likely have a recliner for visitors and a portable table that can be wheeled over to your bed. This is where the delicious hospital food will go.

Your family will be invited in as soon as you are all set up, and the physician will follow shortly after unless an immediate intervention is required. In that case, your physician would have been among the initial welcoming committee.

> ***ICU Confidential Am I Kidnapped Edition:*** If you are confused and agitated and a danger to yourself or others, for example when coming to after sedation, you may find yourself in physical restraints. These are used as a last resort and may include soft ties around your wrists that limit arm movements. Once you are able to fully wake up and are no longer disoriented, you will typically no longer need these restraints and they will be removed. This is why we also try and have family at the bedside, so that you have someone you trust and recognize to re-orient you and remind you that you are safe.

B. The Flow of the ICU

The ICU is truly the city that never sleeps. There's always something going on, and there is an ebb and flow to the daily routine. The following describes a typical day.

The day at the ICU starts early in the morning, at about 5 or 6 am. This is where the various technicians come around and do their thing, like drawing blood and taking X-rays. Why so early? It's so the lab results are available, and the X-ray is up in time for the physicians to have them when we make our rounds.

The mornings are busy with doctors too, especially if you have medical students, residents, and fellows check in on you and do their assessments (6-7 am). This is when **sedation vacations** and decisions regarding **ventilator weaning** happen (more on what this means in Chapter 8: Life Support in the ICU). Nurses typically switch off at 7 am, where the night shift gives report to the day shift. This is a critical time for nursing, so visitation may be limited.

For the physician teams, the medical and specialty rounds follow. This is where the main physician teams come around to evaluate you and make plans for the day (typically 7 am – 11 am). The rest of our day commences with procedures, **extubations, intubations**, scans, IV therapies, family meetings, medical emergencies (**codes**), and more. The team usually splits up and divides new admissions, procedures, discharges, and other responsibilities. When lunch comes around to you, we are also trying to eat if we have time, usually during a lecture, after which the flow resumes until dinner.

All throughout the day, new patients are being admitted to the ICU and improving patients are being transitioned to lower intensity levels of care. Emergencies can elbow their way into the schedule anytime. As evening approaches, elective procedures wind down, and planned extubations become less common. Fewer subspecialists are physically in the hospital and **supportive care** is king, as opposed to making big clinical moves.

Nighttime starts when the day shift nurses sign out and the night shift signs in (typically 7 pm). This is when most ICU physician teams also change shifts. Some hospitals conduct evening rounds where the physician team does a more detailed walk-through on everyone in the ICU.

Patients have a higher threshold to get extubated and have fewer elective procedures done overnight as, again, less becomes more. The ICU physician (and/or house staff) is usually quite busy with new admissions while also addressing any emergencies in the ICU. Sometimes they cover issues in the general wards as well. Physician staffing is typically much lower at night.

Patients are left alone as best as can be done in an ICU to get some sleep. This is often difficult as emergencies don t follow the clock or hospital quiet hours. As morning approaches, the cycle repeats itself.

C. Medical and Specialty Rounds

A typical ICU team, or **multidisciplinary team rounds**, consists of the attending physician, the ICU nurse, the house staff (fellow, residents, interns, and medical students), the physician extender (nurse practitioner or physician assistant), the ICU pharmacist and their students, and sometimes the charge nurse. Respiratory therapy and others round out the team. This can get really big if in a full academic center, and so teams are often split. In most non-academic centers, an ICU team may only include the attending physician who drops in sometime in the morning and is usually accompanied by the nurse and nurse practitioner.

The typical presentation with house staff includes the intern or resident (or sometimes the medical student) presenting your case. This begins with a synopsis of why you are there, a recounting of overnight events, a presentation of your physical exam, labs and imaging findings, and finally the plan for the day. The senior members of the team chime in, as well as nursing, respiratory therapy, and pharmacy, and final decisions are made with the attending.

The team then comes into your room and the attending confirms certain aspects of your history and physical exam. The team adjusts recommendations based on any new information and discusses the plan for the day with you. Teaching is interlaced throughout the rounds.

If you are in a non-academic setting, the ICU physician usually consults the nurse and the chart and says a quick hello to you and goes over the day's plan.

Subspecialty services like cardiology, nephrology, GI and others will usually see you in the morning as well. If there is a fellow or resident, or a physician extender, they will see you pretty early on their own and come back with their whole team.

> ***ICU Confidential More Helpful Tips Edition:*** It's very useful to have your loved ones at your bedside during rounds. This allows you and them to hear updates, explanations, and plans for your care together, leaving less chance for miscommunication and more chance for efficiency. Some physicians will even have you and your family listen in on and even participate in rounds (although this is rare). When we come in to discuss things during rounds, please also include anyone you want to participate from the beginning (including by phone).

> ***ICU Confidential You've Skipped Me Edition:*** You are usually seen based on location, but often the very sickest patients get seen first as decisions may need to be made right away. This also includes emergency procedures like intubations and central line placements. Please don't feel bad if the team initially walks right by your room – it's usually a good sign (for you), and they will be back later.

D. Procedures

Most urgent procedures get done as you are being admitted to the ICU – think surgeries, intubation, **central lines, arterial lines**, and **dialysis** catheters. An acute worsening of your medical condition may also trigger these urgent additional interventions.

If your procedure is not urgent, it usually gets done after rounds. The team divides the work once a full list is compiled. If you are sedated and on a ventilator, we get consent from your medical **power of attorney** (for details, see Chapter 10: Code Status Definitions and Difficult Decisions), and you wouldn't even know it happened. If you are awake and have the capacity to make decisions, we get consent from you and provide sedation depending on the procedure.

Central lines and arterials lines are generally placed by the intern or resident or physician extender. Intubations are done by the attending with the fellow, the respiratory therapist, or a specialist (anesthesiologist if your intensivist isn't one already). If it's an emergency and after hours in a facility without round-the-clock intensivist coverage, the ER or the hospital code team physician performs any emergency procedures.

> ***ICU Confidential How Many of These Have You Done Edition:*** Depending on how your ICU is staffed, most procedures will be performed by a physician extender, be it a nurse practitioner or a resident physician. They are typically very experienced and are doing these procedure on a daily basis. If they are earlier in their career, they will be supervised by a more experienced member of the team. The attending may be very hands on, but usually does procedures much less frequently. In ICUs where you only have a full-time intensivist, they will likely be doing the procedure directly. Either way, you are always within your right to inquire about levels of experience and ask about supervision.

E. Meals

Meals come at regular times if you are eating. The type of diet usually matches your condition (i.e. cardiac diet or renal [kidney] diet). This may be interrupted if you are expecting a procedure or test that requires you not to be eating (“**nil per os**,” or **NPO**). Sometimes, eating happens through a tube in your nose or mouth going directly into your stomach (**gastric tube**). These are tube feeds that have all the nutritional value you will need. We can also use these gastric tubes to deliver medications you would otherwise have to swallow.

> ***ICU Confidential Eating Can Wait Edition:*** Medically speaking, your body can go without food for around 7 days, as long as we keep you hydrated and keep your electrolytes in check. While we try to start feeding you as soon as possible, keep this in mind as there are situations where feeding can be dangerous (high dose medications for low blood pressure, ileus [gut won't work], severe confusion). Sometimes eating does get left behind as we work hard to keep you alive, so if it's been a while, kindly remind us – nutrition is absolutely key to your long-term recovery.

F. Bathrooms

This gets tricky to say the least. If you are entirely bed-ridden, you may have a catheter in your bladder, and a **rectal tube**. If there's no catheter, and you are confined to bed, you may need to go in a bed pan or hand-held urinal. If you are allowed to get up, a bedside commode, like a portable toilet with no walls, is made available. If you have the all clear to go further there are usually toilets that fold out of the cabinets of the ICU (coming soon to Ikea®), or even actual bathrooms attached to your room. Inevitably, we will walk in on you in these private moments. It's almost like we're waiting until you have to go.

> ***ICU Confidential Gotta (Let) Go Edition:*** It's normal to feel like you want to urinate when a catheter is in the bladder, just relax and let go as best you can. You can request a condom or wicker pad catheter that is non-invasive but hopefully still gets the job done. Most high-quality ICUs have some form of catheter rounds so they can identify patients who don't absolutely need them and have them removed before they cause infection. Don't be afraid to speak up and remind the team.

ICU Confidential No Food No Poop Edition: We get this question all the time: I haven't eaten anything so how am I expected to have bowel movements. In fact, you constantly have secretions and mucus, along with sloughing of the cells in your GI tract, and tube feeds that may be going. Your poop may be expected to decrease but does not stop completely. Even if it slows down considerably, you should at least be passing gas to indicate the gut is working.

G. Visitation

ICU visitation hours vary, but they tend to be liberal during the day. Exceptions include during nurse shift changes (around 7 am and 7 pm), and overnight. Most ICUs have a limit of 2 people at a time in the room, no children below a certain age, and no one actively sick (coughing, sneezing, runny nose). No animals either (even if they are better behaved than some adults). Fresh cut flowers are also avoided due to mold and allergies. Overnight hours are usually limited but can be allowed by special arrangement. Because having family at the bedside is well recognized as beneficial to your recovery, we make every effort to maximize this time.

Please be respectful of the rules of your ICU, including keeping the noise down, putting on gowns or gloves when asked, and sanitizing hands before and after room entry. And don't forget the masks when asked. Exceptions to numbers and times are often made when the patient is actively passing away or transitioning to hospice.

ICU Confidential Secret Mission Editon: I've worked in a place where the chief unit physician (allegedly) smuggled in a dying patient's Bichon Frise in a tote bag because of how important this was to the patient. The patient was technically out of the ICU and in inpatient hospice, but this was still against the rules. I instantly became a fan of this Hallmark® channel worthy operation. We can definitely make adjustments, especially during end-of-life care, so ask (nicely and without expectations) – if it's important to you, we will do our best to accommodate; if it's dangerous or inappropriate, we will let you know.

7 Medical Journeys by Diagnosis

As healthcare professionals, when we discuss a patient's list of medical problems, we can do so using two general approaches. The first involves asking what specific medical issues we are treating, categorized by diagnosis. This works well when you have only one or two major health issues, like if you have pneumonia or a heart attack, as it helps us focus our evaluation.

If your problems are broader or systemic, then we may prefer to group your health issues by organ systems, like respiratory and cardiac. In this second way of approaching your medical situation, each organ system gets its own assessment and plan.

This chapter breaks down some of the most common afflictions by diagnosis, keeping in mind that each problem can affect more than one organ.

A. Pneumonia

Pneumonia means you have inflammation in the air sacs of the lungs along with the airways that bring air to and from those air sacs. The most common cause of pneumonia is infection, which starts with being exposed to someone already sick and breathing in the virus or bacteria that they just coughed out. If the infection settles in the airways only, we call this **bronchitis** – similar symptoms but not as severe or dangerous.

When the air sacs get inflamed, they fill up with body fluids consisting of immune response cells and other byproducts like phlegm, immune products, and bacteria and/or viruses. These products of inflammation will plug up the airways if not coughed up and will turn what is normally air-filled alveolar sacs surrounded by small blood vessels into a wet sponge incapable of exchanging oxygen for carbon dioxide (what the lungs are supposed to do).

Aside from infection, pneumonia can also be caused by contact with caustic substances like aspirated food particles and stomach acid, smoke inhalation, and chemicals in the air It can also result from your own immune system attacking the lungs either as a complication of medications, trauma, or from autoimmune diseases.

i. Symptoms

Pneumonia usually causes shortness of breath, a lot of phlegm, and increased cough as the lungs try to clear out all that debris. Sometimes the phlegm can also be blood tinged. Fortunately, cough is one of the strongest and most coordinated physical miracles that your muscles can perform and can widely disperse the used air in your lungs (and all the gross stuff in it) out of your mouth at better than 50 mph. (This is why coughing people are so infectious to all their neighbors and are universally shunned in elevators and airplanes.)

If enough of the airways are impacted by inflammation, you lose more and more of your lung reserve until you get air hunger with less and less activity, and eventually even at rest. Fever, general fatigue and malaise caused by infection, as well as by constant coughing, add to your misery.

Except for the muscle pain you get from coughing, chest pain is not very common in pneumonia because the lungs primarily have pressure and cough receptors, not pain receptors. The lining of the lungs (the **pleura**) is exquisitely sensitive, however, and sometimes inflammation can spread to the outside of the lung causing sharp pain with breathing. This is called **pleurisy** and can sometimes persist well after the infection has passed.

ii. Types

Pneumonias are classified by what causes them and how you acquired them as this has implications for how they are treated.

a. Community Acquired Pneumonia (CAP)

CAP is the typical infection you get while living your normal life outside of the healthcare setting (thanks, community!). It starts with being exposed to someone already sick and breathing on you. If caught early, it can often be treated at home with rest and hydration, and antimicrobial medications if needed.

Often, pneumonia is caused by **viruses** (influenza, Covid, respiratory syncytial virus [RSV], and many more), but **bacteria** also cause community acquired pneumonia (pneumococcus, Hemophilus, mycoplasma, legionella, and others). If the infection becomes severe enough, you see a doctor, and you may even end up in the hospital. If your oxygen levels are really low and you are in distress, you go to the ICU.

b. Hospital Acquired / Health Care Associated Pneumonia (HCAP)

The hospital or nursing home environment has its own types of bacteria that hang out there. Given the extensive use of antibiotics, and patients who may have other predisposing illnesses, these bacteria tend to be different in types and levels of resistance to antibiotics. If you get pneumonia more than 3 or so days after being in a hospital or health care facility, or with a history of recent hospitalizations and IV antibiotic use, you are at much greater risk to be infected with one of these 'professional" microbes. We call them **multi-drug resistant (MDR) bacteria**. These require a different set of antibiotics that may need to be given intravenously and can be more difficult to treat.

c. Ventilator Associated Pneumonia (VAP)

When breathing through a tube in your throat connected to a ventilator, you are at much higher risk for developing pneumonia. One reason is that you no longer have the clearance mechanisms meant to protect you from infection as you can't effectively cough with that tube in your throat. There are also other factors that make you more susceptible, no matter how good your respiratory care is. If you develop pneumonia after 2 or 3 days of being on a ventilator, you are defined as having a VAP. This is treated with antibiotics like those of the hospital acquired type. The best way to prevent VAPs is to get off the ventilator as soon as safely possible, another reason why this is a quality marker.

d. Aspiration pneumonia

When you swallow food or liquids or even your own saliva, a complex set of mechanisms control your throat muscles to move the contents from your mouth to your stomach. Food must travel past the entrance to your trachea which is covered by a movable flap of tissue called the **epiglottis** protecting the closed vocal cords. Food then proceeds down the esophagus and into the stomach.

If you have a swallowing impairment because of stroke, drug overdose, confusion, or intrinsic problem with your swallowing mechanism, you may be at risk for food and liquids taking the wrong exit and entering the windpipe (**trachea**). This usually triggers a cough and out goes the material.

Sometimes, the aspiration can be massive where you can't cough it all out, or insidious like a slowly dripping faucet where the contents trickle down and cause chronic inflammation. You may end up in the ICU as a result of a massive aspiration where stomach contents are thrown up and saturate the airways of the lungs instead of going out of your mouth. A massive aspiration can clog your airways and cause significant inflammation, leading to pneumonia and sometimes requiring a ventilator.

ICU Confidential Can't Stop Won't Stop Edition: You can have a tube going through your mouth or nose directly into the stomach to deliver liquid food (**tube feeds**), but contrary to expectations, this does not prevent aspiration. This is also true for tubes that go through your abdomen directly into your stomach (**percutaneous endoscopic gastrostomy** or **PEG** tube, See Appendix I: Machines and Things). Tube feeds can still accumulate in the stomach and then be vomited up and into the lungs. The secretions from your mouth and throat constantly migrating down can also detour into the lungs. This is why feeding tubes are not appropriate if the primary goal is to avoid chronic aspiration.

e. Auto-immune Pneumonia

Your immune system defends you against infections, but it can attack you as well. This is called **auto-immune** disease, and examples include joint destruction in rheumatoid arthritis, or skin damage in psoriasis. There are also auto-immune conditions where the immune system attacks the lungs and can mimic an infection. This type of pneumonia can also be triggered by certain medications including immunotherapy drugs for cancer. Auto-immune pneumonias are rare, often require additional testing to identify, and are treated with anti-inflammatory medications rather than anti-microbials.

f. Lung Contusion

Inflammation from lung bruising after chest trauma (**contusion**) can lead to pneumonia as well. Lungs can bruise like other organs after trauma resulting in bleeding and severe inflammation.

g. Septic emboli

Rarely, when bacteria are actively circulating in your blood stream, they can seed different parts of the lungs. This can be seen in special circumstances like when you have a weakened immune system or are infected with atypical pathogens (think IV drug users injecting drugs mixed with dirty tap water into the blood stream).

iii. Testing

You may be diagnosed with pneumonia with typical symptoms and a chest X-ray or CT scan showing inflammation in the lungs. To find out the type, samples of phlegm are often collected for culture and additional testing. More recently, testing looks at molecular or chemical fingerprints of the most common viruses and bacteria in addition to growing them in a culture. This helps identify culprits like influenza and Covid-19 right away so appropriate therapy can start quickly.

Sometimes, you do have to depend on cultures which can take days to grow. Antibiotics are started as soon as we suspect infection, and identifying the organism allows us to narrow the antibiotics to the specific bacteria or virus once we have those results. Testing the blood and other body fluids can also identify common bacteria like pneumococcus, legionella, and others.

> ***ICU Confidential Multiple Organisms Edition:*** If a culture result comes back with many different types of organisms it usually means that the sample is contaminated, or that there is no true bacterial infection. This often happens in sputum cultures where the initial result suggests multiple organisms but the final result just states "normal respiratory flora." This likely represents the milieu of different organisms living happily in your mouth and upper respiratory passages, and not a true infection. When an organism is causing pneumonia, it usually outperforms all the other bacteria and is the only one that grows in the culture. This may not apply to wound infections, which can be mixed.

iv. Complications

When infection starts to overwhelm your ability to breathe, you require oxygen and then additional respiratory support while the infection hopefully runs its course. Sometimes that means a machine that breathes for you (**ventilator**, Appendix I: Machines and Things). If the infection gets out of control, you have **sepsis** (see Section C below).

Another common complication is the accumulation of fluid outside the lungs but inside the chest cavity. If you think of the chest as a barrel with two partially inflated balloons filling up the space (the lungs), and you add water to the barrel, it collapses the balloons out of the way. This fluid is called a **pleural effusion**. It can develop from lots of other sources, but pneumonia is on the list. This fluid can get actively infected and not just inflamed and turn into pus (**empyema**) that needs to be urgently drained, often leaving a catheter in the chest until the infection runs its course (see Treatments below).

v. Treatments

Antibiotics and antivirals are the mainstay of therapy. How fast you start antimicrobials has a big impact on your survivability. Supportive care with extra oxygen is essential when needed, including progressing to a ventilator if necessary. Non-invasive ventilation (like **BPAP**, see Appendix I, Machines and Things) is not usually a good option as it tends to compact mucus in the airways further without the ability to effectively clear them.

Sometimes, very thick mucus plugs up and collapses an entire part of the lung. This situation can benefit from a **bronchoscopy** where a scope is snaked into your airways for a physical cleanout (see Appendix II: Common Procedures in the ICU). You are usually already on a ventilator for this. Doing a bronchoscopy on most pneumonias is not recommended, as the on-going inflammation from the pneumonia will just replace the mucus you just removed.

If you have a lot of fluid around the lungs, or pleural effusion, it is typically not infected but just inflammatory and will reabsorb on its own as you recover. A procedure called a **thoracentesis** where a needle and catheter are used to remove this fluid and allow that part of the lung to re-expand is sometimes needed. A drain may be left in for a few days to allow any additional fluid to be evacuated (see Appendix II: Common Procedures to Expect in ICU Patients).

In cases of massive aspiration pneumonia, there may be large food particles stuck in the airways that won't come out on their own. Bronchoscopy is then offered to try to retrieve those particles out of your airway through suction and use of specialized tools.

vi. Prevention

The best way to prevent pneumonia is to stay away from sick people, and to stay as healthy as possible (what great advice!). If you have risk factors like having chronic lung disease (COPD, emphysema), or are immunocompromised, being appropriately vaccinated so your immune system is already primed to fight the infection can save your life. This won't prevent infection, but it does give your body the ability to kill these microbial invaders before the infection gets out of control.

If you are at risk for aspiration because of severe confusion, a large upper gastrointestinal bleed, or major trauma, intubation to protect your airway may be required. Identifying what consistency of food you can eat through a swallow study (and sticking to it), as well as eating slowly and in the sitting up position, can help. If you are on a ventilator, having your head of bed elevated at least 30 degrees and getting off the ventilator as soon as possible, as well as getting proper mouth care, will also help prevent those types of pneumonias.

B. Acute Respiratory Distress Syndrome (ARDS):

Acute respiratory distress syndrome is a very serious condition that looks like pneumonia but applies to the entire lungs at the same time. Think about the mechanism of pneumonia as described above, and apply it to both lungs, all at once. ARDS is caused by your own immune system over responding to whatever is triggering inflammation in your body. While it can be triggered by lung infection, any severe infection in the body can cause it (**sepsis**). ARDS can also be triggered by multi-organ failure, severe trauma, and by the stress of being on a ventilator itself. It's important to point out that ARDS can develop in previously healthy people, although it is more common in patients who are already critically ill.

Technically, ARDS is defined as having low oxygen levels, having both lungs significantly inflamed as confirmed by a chest X-ray or CT scan, and *not* being caused by congestive heart failure which can show a similar picture. Distinguishing it from heart failure is important because the lung fluid from heart failure is not inflammatory and is treated with different medications (like **diuretics**, or medications that make you urinate).

i. Symptoms

ARDS makes it hard to breathe. As it progresses, more fluid saturates your lungs making breathing difficult even at rest. As with pneumonia, you may develop a cough with frothy clear or white mucus. As your chest-Xray or CT scan begins to look worse (whitening or opacification representing fluid build-up), you develop higher oxygen requirements and worsening air hunger.

ii. Complications

Aside from all the complications of having to go on a ventilator, the main complication is dying. ARDS is as serious as it gets with a mortality rate of over 45%. If it doesn't kill you, it often makes you weaker due to the need for prolonged ventilator support, and may progress to chronic scarring of the lungs (**fibrosis**). Fortunately, your lungs, like most of your organs, have a lot of reserve built in, and with time and therapy, recovery is possible.

iii. Treatment

We treat the underlying trigger, but specific treatment for ARDS is largely supportive, designed to enable the inflammatory process to run its course without killing you. This means supporting your oxygen levels, including with a ventilator if needed (and it often is). Your lungs are in a delicate situation, so we need to carefully help them do their job of getting you the oxygen you need while avoiding damaging them more than they already are.

We use specific ventilator strategies that baby the lungs by keeping the air pressure low and avoiding both over inflating them and *over*-oxygenating them. It's a fine line, providing enough support to keep you alive, but not too much that the ARDS worsens. Sometimes, we administer steroids or other anti-inflammatory medications.

When all else fails, and you are otherwise young(ish) (that is, have good survivability), we can offer **extracorporeal membrane oxygenation (ECMO)** to oxygenate your blood by bypassing your lungs completely (see Appendix II: Common Procedures in the ICU). ECMO works best if initiated early. If your lungs are beyond recovery, and you meet about 1001 criteria for survivability, a **lung transplant** is the ultimate option.

C. Sepsis

The technical definition of sepsis is a dysregulated host immune response to infection. Translated, this means that in trying to fight off infection, your immune system goes out of control (becomes dysregulated) which causes a lot of collateral damage Think of your immune system as an army putting down an invasion, except instead of just killing the attackers, it starts to set fire to and destroy its own cities and infrastructure. This starts a cascade of problems that can lead to organ failure, blood pressure collapse (**shock**), and death. If you are septic and your blood pressure drops too low, your mortality rate jumps to over 40%, which is higher than dying from a major stroke or heart attack.

i. Symptoms and Sources

While specific symptoms of sepsis vary based on the source of infection, sepsis itself makes you very tired. You tend to lose your appetite and just feel drained. Fevers and sweats are common. Confusion is extremely common, especially in older patients. In fact, confusion and fatigue are often the first and only symptoms in older patients right before they go into shock and try to die, so a sepsis diagnosis is always on our radar (have a high suspicion, treat immediately).

Different microorganisms are known to cause infections in different organs, so treatment is geared towards the organ or site causing infection.

a. Lungs (Pneumonia)

Infection of the lungs is a common source of sepsis. Pneumococcus (also called streptococcus) is the most common bacterial cause, with haemophilus influenza (not to be confused with the influenza virus), staphylococcus aureus, and Legionella also common. Viral causes include Influenza (virus), rhinovirus (common cold gone bad), respiratory syncytial virus (RSV), and coronavirus (including Covid-19). Pneumonia is described as its own medical journey above.

b. Urinary Tract and Kidneys (Urosepsis)

Bacterial infections of the urinary track (bladder and kidneys) tend to have a special talent for progressing to sepsis. A particular group of microbes called **gram-negative bacteria** tends to spread quickly through the bladder and into the kidneys and blood stream. These include E. Coli, Proteus, Klebsiella, Enterobacter, and Pseudomonas. Urosepsis is very inflammatory and can take you from feeling a little tired to needing the ICU in a span of hours. Painful, low volume, dark, and smelly urine are common signs. Pain on tapping the sides at the level of the lower back (**costophrenic tenderness**) can be a sign that the infection has spread to the kidneys (**pyelonephritis**). Having a urinary catheter, kidney stone, or having prior surgery with anatomic abnormalities of the urinary system can predispose you to this type of infection.

c. GI sources

An infection anywhere along your gastrointestinal track can progress to sepsis. Common sites of infection are the gallbladder (**cholangitis**), liver (**hepatitis**), pancreas, and small and large intestines (**gastroenteritis**). "Bad" bacteria in the gut can overwhelm the "good" bacteria and cause significant inflammation as well. This allows them to cross into the blood stream (**translocation**) and trigger sepsis. Symptoms usually include abrupt abdominal pain, diarrhea, and changes in bowel habits.

A particularly nasty GI infection is caused by Clostridioides difficile (**C. diff**). Taking antibiotics for other infections can wipe out the good bacteria in the gut and allow C. diff to blossom and cause severe infection. Unrelenting diarrhea with a particular smell is usually seen. Only a few antibiotics are able to clear a C. diff infection, often requiring a prolonged course of treatment. C. diff infection is extremely contagious, which is why barrier protection (those cool plastic suits) and frequent washing with soap and water (hand sanitizers don't kill C. diff) are so important.

d. Line Sepsis

Patients that have indwelling catheters (we refer to them as **lines**) while in the hospital or who need them as outpatients for chronic treatments like dialysis, chemotherapy, or long-term antibiotics, are susceptible to infections from these catheters. Bacteria can migrate along the surface of or through the catheter itself into the soft tissues and cause local and blood stream infections. The longer you have the catheter, and the closer it is to less sanitary parts of your body (the groin, for example), the greater the risk.

To reduce the risk of line sepsis, we (and you) need to practice excellent catheter hygiene and careful monitoring for signs of infection. In addition, having a **tunneled catheter** that is designed so that a sizable portion of its length lies just under the skin before accessing the blood vessel, can decrease the chance of infection. This is why most home catheters meant for long term use are tunneled. The best protection, however, is not having the catheter in the first place, or getting it removed as soon as you no longer need it (this is a quality measure in most ICUs).

e. Wound Infections:

Traumatic or surgical wounds need special care and attention. Diabetic foot ulcers are a common source of infections that can lead to sepsis. The use of dressings, proper wound care, and specialized devices like wound vacuums all decrease the chance of infection. Sometimes, surgical debridement where dead or necrotic tissue is surgically removed is needed as well. Culturing wounds can be useful, but wounds can also have a cocktail of different bacteria with difficulty telling the bystander (colonizer) from the one causing the infection.

f. Fungal Infections:

A fungus in your bloodstream is called **fungemia**. Fungal organisms are typically very well defended against by our immune systems, much better than against most bacteria. If you get this type of infection, it means either the immune system is weakened, or the type of fungus is particularly strong. A bloodborne fungal infection very often turns into sepsis. People who are immunocompromised (on chemotherapy, have an autoimmune disease, or HIV/AIDS) are at increased risk. Being fed through a central IV line, called **TPN** or **total parenteral nutrition**, is also a risk factor. Treating systemic fungal infections requires an extensive search for the source and long-term administration of anti-fungal medications.

g. Unknown Source:

Up to 30% (yes, THIRTY PERCENT) of the time, the body enters a state of sepsis with an unclear source of infection. This is often true in patients with severe immunodeficiency, or who are chronically ill and frail, but can also be seen in previously healthy people. Sometimes, even if micro-organisms are cultured from the blood stream, their origin can remain a mystery. You are typically given very broad antimicrobials until the source can be narrowed down when more targeted medications can be administered.

ii. Testing:

If we suspect that you have sepsis, we get an array of **cultures** which include samples of blood, sputum, urine, and other bodily fluids. The samples are sent to the microbiology lab where they are subjected to chemical and DNA testing for specific common organisms. They are also left to marinate in special food to see if any microorganisms grow (culture). The body fluids we sample are typically sterile so nothing should grow when they are cultured. If something does, then we have our culprit.

In truth, however, these samples can be contaminated from the needle if the skin is not thoroughly cleaned before the blood draw, or the sputum can include some of the bacteria from the mouth and not the actual lung. Cultures can also take days to grow, so we don't wait to treat you until we have a result because without treatment, you could get much sicker or die from overwhelming infection by then.

Once an organism is identified, it is tested against typical antibiotics known to be effective, yielding an **antibiotic sensitivity panel** that helps guide the choice of antibiotic to give you. There are also chemical and DNA tests designed to look for molecular or genetic traces that can suggest which antibiotics will work best.

There are also a number of really great test arrays that within an hour or less tell you if you have influenza, Covid-19, RSV, and dozens of other viruses. The same is in the works for common bacterial infections. These use advanced technologies for looking at genetic or chemical markers specific to certain microorganisms. There are also some blood and urine tests that help identify immune responses specific for pneumococcus (the most common bacterial cause of pneumonia), Legionella, mycoplasma, and more, yielding results in minutes/hours, rather than days.

> ***ICU Confidential Culture Wars Edition:*** Culture results rarely identify something that's not already being treated with the initial shotgun antibiotic approach we use. Their main benefit is to enable us to use fewer antibiotics since we then know exactly what to target. Cultures may grow nothing at all, even when there is an obvious infection. This is a limitation of the test and does necessarily mean there's no infection. Cultures also help us identify bacteria that are resistant to certain antibiotics and again allow us to target them more precisely. So, while culture results are important in guiding how we care for you, they must be interpreted in the context of everything else going on.

In addition to looking for micro-organisms, we also gauge how sick you are with several labs indicating degree of inflammation or "panic" in your body. This may include checking your **white blood cell count**, **procalcitonin** level, and more. To see how starved your organs are of proper blood supply (shock), we check a **lactate** level.

iii. Complications

The most severe complication of sepsis is very low blood pressure (shock) that starves the organs of their oxygen and nutrient supply leading to **multi-organ failure** and death. Complications are common to the site of infection, like respiratory failure for pneumonia, kidney failure in urosepsis, and so forth. Confusion and overwhelming fatigue are also common.

Even when sepsis is effectively treated, it can be complicated by weakness and prolonged recovery because of being laid up in bed and not eating. Specific organs may not fully recover, most commonly kidney failure needing dialysis. Getting sepsis, like many critical illnesses, is kind of like getting hit by a truck. You may get up and limp away, but it can be a long road to recovery.

iv. Treatment

Perhaps the most important part of treating sepsis is recognizing it in the first place. Several check lists are used to help the clinician recognize sepsis early and often. These markers include changes to your **vital signs** (fever, low blood pressure, rapid heart rate, low oxygen level), and signs of organ damage (blood tests for kidney function, liver function, and so on).

The mainstay of treatment is beginning antibiotics right away. In fact, this quality marker is so important that the hospital is hit with a financial penalty if antibiotics are delayed. As antibiotics are going in, your health care team is searching for what is causing the sepsis, what we call **source control**. Is it an abscess, a gallstone, or an infected catheter in your bladder? Is it an infected kidney stone? As soon as possible, this problem must be remedied.

At the same time as we are starting antibiotics, we rehydrate you and stay ahead of any blood pressure drop, a common phenomenon in sepsis. This is called **fluid resuscitation** (not to be confused with the other type of resuscitation such as CPR.) Our magic number for how much IV fluid to give is currently 30 ml of intravenous fluid per kg of body weight, administered over the first three hours. For a 220 lb person, this is about 3 liters (or the better part of a gallon). Often, much more fluid is needed, as are adrenalin-like IV medications (**pressors**) to keep your blood pressure up (we discuss details in Chapter 8: Life Support in the ICU, and in Appendix III: Medications in the ICU).

If, despite the fluids and IV medications, the blood pressure remains too low, we call this refractory septic shock, or big trouble. In summary, Recognize, Antibiotics, Resuscitate – RAR!

D. Heart Attacks, Arrhythmias, and Congestive Heart Failure

The heart is the main driver of circulation of blood throughout the body. It is a complex muscle with 4 chambers all working together to circulate blood. The role of the right side of the heart is to receive oxygen-poor carbon-dioxide-rich blood from the body into the right atrium and pump it into the lungs through the right ventricle. Oxygen is absorbed into and carbon dioxide is released out of the blood in the lungs, and the "refreshed" blood returns to the heart into the left atrium. It then travels to the left ventricle, the workhorse of the heart, where it gets pumped into the aorta and distributed throughout the body.

When the heart fails, the delivery of oxygen and nutrients starts to decrease, and organs start to struggle. The heart can fail when the muscle or valves aren't working, or the coordination (**rhythm**) isn't right.

i. Symptoms

When the heart is failing, whether due to a part of the muscle not working properly or the whole thing not beating rhythmically, multiple symptoms can occur (like in your favorite country song). The following summarizes these symptoms and how they come about:

a. Heart Attacks aka Acute Myocardial Infarction aka Acute Coronary Syndrome

Is it a widow maker or just that burrito from lunch? The classic symptoms of a heart attack include chest pressure with radiation to the neck and down the left arm, shortness of breath, sweating, and an overall feeling of doom. But there are definitely more subtle presentations. Sometimes, just feeling tired or having what you think is indigestion can signal worse things to come.

If you get symptoms with physical activity, or eventually even at rest, we call this **angina**, an important warning sign. Patients with diabetes and women are more likely not to have the typical presentation. If you have risk factors, please speak with your primary care physician and get the right outpatient testing. If symptoms are worsening and you're in doubt, get medical care right away. It's better to burp your way to feeling better in the ER than to die of a heart attack at home.

b. Arrhythmias

These refer to any abnormality in the *lub-dub* rhythm the heart normally makes. The 4 chambers of the heart pump in sequence with a cadence that changes according to the body's needs, relying on a specialized electrical (conductance) system to control this. When this system fails and the heart no longer beats together, or beats in an irregular way, we call this an **arrhythmia**.

Arrhythmias come in different types, from a problem in the atria (for example, **atrial fibrillation**), to a problem in the ventricles (**ventricular fibrillation**). It can beat too fast (**tachycardia**) or too slow (**bradycardia**). An arrhythmia that is serious enough to cause low blood pressure and related symptoms can quickly become dangerous. That palpitation you felt may be the triple espresso, or it may be an arrhythmia that needs immediate attention.

One of the most common arrhythmias in the ICU, and for outpatients, is **atrial fibrillation**, or **afib** for short (not a lie). It can be triggered by almost any stress on your body, including being in the ICU for any reason. The upper chambers of the heart (the atria) start to quiver instead of contracting to a regular beat. This can cause the whole heart to contract in an irregular way and sometimes beat dangerously fast, making you very uncomfortable and severely lowering your blood pressure. Afib can be controlled with medications, or if you're unstable, with an electric shock (**cardioversion**). Afib can also increase your long-term risk for blood clots and so you may require a blood thinner (**anticoagulation**).

c. Congestive Heart Failure:

If the pump starts to fail, whether because of arrhythmias or weakened heart muscle, the circulation of blood throughout the body decreases. It leads to swelling in the legs and arms (**peripheral edema**), and accumulation of fluid in the lungs (**pulmonary edema**). This makes it harder to breathe as you start drowning in your own fluids. Congestive heart failure is managed by treating the underlying cause as best as possible, and with medications called **diuretics** which work on the kidneys to make you urinate out more fluid (or dialysis if your kidneys don't work).

ii. Evaluation

In evaluating you for heart problems, we start by measuring your **vital signs** as we ask you specific questions about your symptoms and your medical history. We draw blood and get an **EKG** and a **chest X-ray.** The blood tests include checking markers of heart muscle damage (for example, **troponin** increases with heart muscle damage, and **pro-BNP** increases with heart failure) along with your electrolytes, kidney and liver function (**comprehensive metabolic panel**, or **CMP**), and general counts of the different types of blood cells (**complete blood count**, or **CBC**).

We perform an electrocardiogram (EKG or ECG) by placing some sensors on your chest and limbs. The sensors pick up the heart's electrical activity and show us a pattern that may suggest a specific heart problem. An EKG not only shows arrhythmias but also shows key changes consistent with on-going heart damage. It allows us to estimate which part of the heart is struggling, and how dangerous this struggle is. If there is concern about an evolving heart attack, it may lead to a slew of medications meant to slow the heart damage, and potentially an emergency procedure called **cardiac catheterization** to open a blocked coronary artery and stop the heart attack.

iii. To Cath or Not to Cath?

The main determination of the danger of a heart attack is how much of the heart muscle is affected. If it looks like the muscle is starved for blood through its entire width, we call this an **ST Elevation MI (STEMI)** referring to the type of change we see on the EKG. This is a cardiac emergency that has a high chance of killing you if not addressed right away. The standard of care is to go to the **catheterization laboratory (cath lab)** right away.

In the cath lab, a catheter is fed into an artery (often in the wrist or groin) and passed into the arteries supplying your heart (coronary arteries). Using this catheter, dye is injected directly into the coronary arteries to identify blockages that can be opened with a balloon (**angioplasty**). A **coronary stent** may be deployed to keep the blockage from recurring (see Appendix II: Common Procedures in the ICU for more details).

If your facility doesn't offer catheterizations and the closest hospital that does will take too long to get to, you can also receive a heavy-duty blood thinner or clot buster as an alternative If the EKG shows only partial damage to the heart muscle (ST depression MI, or **non-STEMI**) a trip to the cath lab is a judgement call. In those situations, the first option is to stabilize your heart with medication before going to the lab.

> ***ICU Confidential Call for Backup Edition:*** There are circumstances when your coronary artery anatomy is very complex, including if you've had prior angioplasty and stents, or when we already know you have blockages in areas that are very difficult to get to using a catheter. In these situations, it is important to have surgical back-up in case the cardiac cath is not able to fix the problem. Patients many need to go from the cath lab straight to the operating room for **coronary artery bypass surgery** (**CABG**), and it's important to be in a facility that has this readily available.

iv. More Help is on the Way

A number of higher-level heart failure therapies are available in more specialized centers. Advanced medications, intra-aortic balloon pumps, and other invasive devices can be added to support (see Appendix I: Machines and Things for more, but only if you want to). Pacemakers can become necessary to help certain arrhythmias. This may be combined with an automatic implantable cadioverter defibrilator (**AICD**) to prevent fatal arrhythmias. As noted above, in cases where the coronary vessels are not able to be fixed, coronary artery bypass graft (CABG) surgery may be required.

E. Kidney Failure

The kidneys not only filter out toxins from the blood stream but also perform other vital bodily functions. They help manage electrolytes, balance the acid-base (**pH**) in your body, and remove excess fluid (turning it to urine) to keep your body fluid levels balanced (**euvolemic**). Kidneys essentially maintain a balanced chemical environment so the normal processes of the body can take place.

Kidney failure is very common in the background of critical illness. Kidney damage can be caused by infection, low blood pressure, as well as from medications and dyes used in medical tests. They can be chronically compromised by diabetes and poorly controlled high blood pressure (**hypertension**). We monitor kidney function through routine blood tests (**creatinine** and **BUN**) and by tracking how much you are urinating. When we detect trouble, we try to determine the cause by testing the urine and blood and sometimes perform an ultrasound of the kidneys.

i. Dialysis

When the kidneys can no longer manage the body's essential chemicals (for example, they can't control the acid-base balance, or pH), or when they can't excrete enough urine and your body starts to swell, then artificially replacing kidney function becomes necessary. This is what we call **dialysis**, or **renal replacement therapy** (**RRT**). Dialysis is the process of removing blood from your body, filtering it through a machine that removes toxins and excess liquid (and can add electrolytes and other chemicals), and returns it to the body in a continuous cycle typically lasting several hours per day.

Dialysis may also be necessary to remove certain poisonings or overdoses of medications. Finally, a form of dialysis can be used to filter out certain immune chemicals in a set of acute auto-immune conditions.

Dialysis is a form of life support in the ICU and receiving it emergently requires a special kind of very large IV catheter called a **dialysis catheter**. This has its own set of complications which need to be considered when deciding whether to give consent. Check out Appendix I: Machines and Things, for more information.

> ***ICU Confidential Chronic Dialysis Edition:*** Long-term dialysis performed for several hours three times a week in a dialysis center or at home is a chronic outpatient therapy used by many individuals. The technology is similar to what you may need in the ICU, but you have a fistula (a surgical connection of blood vessels in your arm; this takes 2-3 months to mature before it can be used) or tunneled catheter for long term use. Urgent dialysis in the ICU is more dangerous as it often occurs in the context of other rapidly evolving health conditions.

> ***ICU Confidential How Slow Can You Go Edition:*** A major side effect of dialysis is a precipitous drop in blood pressure. If your blood pressure is already low, special forms of dialysis can be performed where blood is removed and filtered much more slowly to avoid significant shifts in blood volume. This may require continuous dialysis where you are connected to the dialysis machine around the clock and requires the ICU.

F. Liver Failure

The liver is a detoxification powerhouse. It cleans the blood from certain toxins like ammonia that, if allowed to accumulate, can make you very confused even to the point of going into a coma. The liver also provides the necessary chemicals to keep our blood from becoming too thin causing spontaneous bleeding, produces bile necessary for digestion, and plays a role in immunity as well as protein production.

The liver can acutely fail, or it may fail slowly over months to years. When the liver becomes so scarred that it is unlikely to recover, we call this **cirrhosis**. While there are medications and blood products that can help compensate for a failing liver, presently, the liver cannot be fully replaced with technology. Only a liver transplant can give you a fresh start.

i. Causes and Diagnosis

Viral infections (hepatitis A, B, C and more), intoxications (such as chronic alcohol use, acetaminophen and other drug overdoses), very low blood pressure (shock liver), liver cancer, genetic diseases (e.g. Wilson's disease) and fatty liver disease can all lead to severe liver damage. Diagnosing the cause may be evident from medical history and some basic blood tests, or may require specialized blood tests, and imaging like ultrasound, CT scan, and MRI. Sometimes, a liver biopsy is needed to fully assess the amount of damage and its cause.

ii. Symptoms

Yellowing of the skin and the conjunctiva (the "whites of your eyes" become yellow) is what we call **jaundice** and can occur with certain types of liver disease. The yellowing happens because the damaged liver can no longer process **bilirubin**, a yellow-orange pigment, into bile causing it to accumulate. Abdominal pain, especially in the upper right quadrant, nausea, and vomiting are common symptoms of liver damage. As noted, accumulation of ammonia can lead to confusion and, in severe cases, may put you in a coma.

Easy bruising to brisk bleeding can occur as your blood gets too thin to **coagulate**. Liver failure also leads to excessive protein loss which causes significant fluid retention. This fluid seeps into your abdominal cavity (**ascites**) and chest cavity (**pleural effusion**), and saturates the soft tissues in your legs, arms, and torso (**anasarca**). We call this **third spacing** and it's usually a bad sign.

iii. Complications

There are several serious complications of liver failure when it comes to the ICU. The first is confusion and agitation eventually leading to coma. The confusion can be very severe where you do wildly inappropriate things that make you a danger to yourself and others. It can lead to stupor and coma, and when you can't reliably breathe on your own, intubation for **airway protection** may be required.

The second set of complications has to do with your propensity to bleed. As liver failure worsens, the liver's ability to produce

clotting factors plummets and requires replacement with transfusions of blood products (red blood cells, fresh frozen plasma, cryoprecipitate, platelets), sometimes many units per day. These replace the clotting factors the liver can no longer produce, and blood that you've already lost.

Another source of bleeding in chronic liver disease is abnormal blood vessels in the esophagus (**esophageal varices**). Because a dying liver increases the pressure in the venous system (**portal hypertension**), blood vessels get abnormally dilated to try to decompress this pressure. These can be at the surface of your esophageal lining and are very prone to bleeding. Without improving liver function, this situation only gets worse, and you will have a high chance of severe bleeding.

The third main complication is fluid accumulating in the abdomen and sometimes the chest and soft tissues. Fluid buildup creates pressure in these cavities and tissues, causing severe discomfort. This can make you very short of breath and increases the risk of infection (including in the abdominal fluid, called **spontaneous bacterial peritonitis**, or **SBP**). It can also make it much more dangerous to undergo invasive procedures.

A failing liver puts stress on other organs as well, increasing the risk of kidney failure (**hepato-renal syndrome**) and respiratory failure (**hepato-pulmonary syndrome**). These multi-organ failure scenarios are difficult to manage without being able to fix the liver. When they get bad enough, you will likely require dialysis and/or ventilator support.

iv. Treatments

Depending on the cause of your liver failure, effective treatment may be available. If it's a toxin that we can flush out or counteract, we do it. If it's an infection or an acute immune reaction, we treat it. If it's due to shock, we treat whatever's causing the shock and support you as we give the liver some time to recover.

Unfortunately, many patients end up in the ICU because their liver failure is a chronic issue that's worsened through natural progression of the underlying disease, and this becomes irreversible. There are some medications we can give to support a failing liver and delay complications (rifampin, beta-blockers, diuretics, nutritional support), but ultimately, your only hope may be a liver transplant.

ICU Confidential One For the Road Edition: Taking care of liver patients in the ICU can be very challenging. They are usually dying, sometimes in denial, and have limited treatment options. They are more than likely confused and combative, and they bleed, often profusely, consuming many bags of blood products and making any invasive procedures much riskier. Some are still actively addicted to alcohol. There are, of course, many patients with chronic liver disease not due to alcohol or other addictions. For most patients, liver transplantation is not an option, and they succumb to complications. Either way, our job is to do our best to take care of them and give them every chance to get home to their loved ones again, or to make their passing as comfortable as possible.

ICU Confidential Michelin Person Edition: When the body goes into full swelling mode it's usually an ominous sign that everything is highly inflamed. We can see this in liver failure as discussed above, as well as in kidney failure, but also in general states of severe illness like sepsis, after major surgery, or after severe trauma. This becomes very scary when you see yourself or your loved one become swollen. By the same token, when this swelling starts to clear, it is a very good sign.

G. Stroke / Cerebrovascular Accident (CVA)

The brain is extremely sensitive to loss of blood flow and oxygen. A problem with the blood supply to any part of the brain rapidly damages the affected tissues, which results in potentially catastrophic outcomes. There are two main mechanisms that lead to a stroke, and they are treated very differently.

i. Ischemic (Embolic)

By far the most common type of stroke, an embolism is a blood clot that physically blocks an artery supplying the brain thereby cutting off blood flow. The clot can come from somewhere else in the body (like the heart during an arrhythmia called atrial fibrillation) or it can develop in the affected vessel over time. The part of the brain that is deprived of blood flow (**ischemia**) starts to die. Inflammation and swelling ensue causing additional damage. An ischemic stroke is diagnosed with imaging and treated with blood thinners and potentially catheter-driven interventions like **thrombectomies**, where the clot is removed using very specialized skills.

ii. Hemorrhagic (Bleeding):

Due to trauma, a leaking aneurysm, a brain tumor, a dissection of a blood vessel, or after conversion of a larger embolic stroke, bleeding into the brain is invariably bad news (!). The blood, which is pumped at high pressure relative to the gelatinous brain, compresses the brain against your rigid skull. This, along with the inflammation that occurs with the overly compressed brain cells, results in swelling and further brain damage. Bleeding may occur within the brain tissue itself (common in aneurysm or tumor), or between the brain and the skull (common in trauma).

In very specific situations, it may be possible to stop the bleeding by putting a coil into the bleeding blood vessel with a catheter, thereby clotting it off (done by neurointerventional radiology). In some scenarios, decompressing the skull with burr holes or a **craniotomy** (cutting the skull open, done by neurosurgery) may be indicated. This requires highly specialized centers with advanced expertise and ICU resources.

H. Pulmonary Embolus (PE)

When a blood clot goes into the blood vessels of your lungs and blocks the circulation, that part of the lung is no longer able to absorb oxygen. The blood clot(s) usually develops in the larger veins of your legs (**deep vein thrombosis**, or **DVT**) and travel through the right side of the heart and into the lung circulation. They can break up into smaller clots and occlude multiple blood vessels at the same time.

DVTs and PEs don't usually require the ICU, but if enough vessels get occluded, your oxygen levels drop and you get very short of breath. This can also cause a rapid drop in blood pressure (shock) due to failure of the right ventricle of the heart as it tries to pump against the clogged pipes. This requires rapid intervention with clot busters or mechanical interventions, and close monitoring in the ICU.

Aside from starting a blood thinner, there are several interventions available to help mechanically break up the clot, typically performed by an interventional radiologist or sometimes a vascular surgeon. There is also a chronic version of PEs that can lead to elevated blood pressure in the lung circulation eventually causing major symptoms like shortness of breath and passing out (this is called **pulmonary hypertension**).

I. Cancer...

... doesn't kill you, the complications do. While physical tumors can erode into blood vessels or push on vital organs, the most common complication from cancer is infection leading to sepsis and shock. People with advanced cancer are at particularly high risk for infection because their immune system function diminishes, they may be malnourished and have significant frailty. In addition to infections, other complications from cancer include blood clots, strokes, heart attacks, and organ damage specific to the cancer.

Complications from cancer therapies can be severe as well. The various chemotherapy and immunotherapy drugs, radiation treatments, and cancer surgeries can cause severe complications. They can further degrade your immune system, cause allergic or autoimmune reactions, and be directly toxic to specific organs.

Given enough time, just about every solid cancer will spread through the rest of the body. This is referred to as **metastatic disease**. Different types of cancers tend to metastasize to different parts of the body. With few exceptions, this means that surgical treatment is no longer an option. We see a lot of this in the ICU since by this point patients are at the end stage of their disease.

All the above can make you sick enough to need the ICU. The following includes site-specific complications seen in some of the more common cancers.

i. Central Nervous System (CNS) Tumors

Gliomas are the most common types of CNS tumors and include subtypes like astrocytoma and glioblastoma. Other CNS cancers include meningiomas, CNS lymphoma, and metastatic cancers from other organs. The most common complications of CNS tumors result from the increased pressure the tumors create in the brain. As discussed in strokes above, the brain is encased in a hard shell (the skull), and when there's something growing and/or causing swelling, the brain gets compressed and can no longer function correctly.

Symptoms include headaches, vomiting, and confusion and may require immediate intervention. Other symptoms can be specific to the site of the tumor in the brain, causing weakness of a specific body part, or difficulty talking. We can use steroids and other medications to temporarily decrease swelling, as well as radiation therapy, and sometimes surgical therapies to help relieve the pressure.

ii. Mouth, Throat and Neck Tumors

Solid tumors of the tongue, throat and neck are typically squamous cell carcinomas. These tumors can get bulky and occlude the airway, making breathing difficult and necessitating the ICU. Placing a breathing (**endotracheal**) tube if you need a ventilator becomes harder with a large tumor getting in the way. This may also require using video and/or bronchoscopy for intubation and is best done in a controlled and pre-emptive setting, not in an emergency.

The other major ICU concern with these types of tumors is bleeding. Head and neck tumors tend to be highly vascularized and prone to bleeding. They can ulcerate and cause slow bleeding or can result in a sudden burst blood vessel leading to rapid profuse bleeding. Aside from acute blood loss in a place that may be difficult to compress, the problem is again the airway. When trying to **intubate**, in addition to the physical tumor, we have a sea of red in the camera preventing us from seeing the vocal cords.

Other complications from these tumors include aspirating food and secretions into your lungs, difficulties with your speech, and complications from a tracheostomy tube if you have one.

There are also two important hormone-producing glands in the neck; the thyroid and parathyroid. Cancer (and other factors) affecting these glands can cause significant hormonal dysfunction. In some cases, thyroid hormone levels become dangerously low (**hypothyroidism**) causing **myxedema coma** that results in shock and dangerously low body temperature. In some cases, you can have very high thyroid levels (**thyroid storm**) which can cause dangerously high blood pressure and rapid heart rate. The **parathyroid glands** help regulate calcium levels in the body. When calcium levels become very high or very low, that can also be quite dangerous and require ICU admission.

iii. Lung Cancer

Lung cancers are usually classified as **non-small cell** and **small cell,** based on how the cancer cells look under the microscope. Non-small cell cancers are further classified into subtypes, and they all behave somewhat differently. There are also cancers that affect the lining of the lung, such as mesotheliomas, and (rarely) sarcomas. From an ICU perspective, our main concerns include low oxygen (**hypoxia**), pneumonia, liquid in the chest (**pleural effusion**) and airway bleeding.

a. Airway Obstruction Causing Shortness of Breath:

When a lung mass grows it can push on and/or invade into the airway (**bronchus**) and cut off the air supply to that part of the lung. This can make you short of breath when the rest of the lung can no longer compensate. If the tumor is invading through the airway (or growing from inside it), it can also be prone to bleeding which further obstructs the airway.

b. Post Obstructive Pneumonia:

A lung tumor can reduce your ability to bring up mucus from beyond that obstruction. The lungs have a natural protection and hydration system - a constant production of mucus coating the inside of the airways. This keeps the airways moist and sticky, helping trap particulates and microbes in the air we breathe.

The mucus is constantly being pushed along through what's called a **mucociliary escalator**. Tiny hair-like projections coating the inside of the airways move in a coordinated fashion to "row" the mucus out of the smaller airway and eventually into the windpipe (**trachea**) and then out of the lungs.

When this process is disrupted by an obstructing tumor, the mucus builds up and creates a perfect breeding ground for infection. This triggers production of even more mucus and sometimes pus that can't easily be coughed up. This is called post-obstructive pneumonia and can be severe enough to require the ICU.

c. Airway Bleeding:

The erosion of blood vessels as the tumor grows can result in profuse bleeding into the airway. Blood can fall further into the bronchus filling it completely. It can also come up towards the windpipe and spill over to other airways plugging them up as well. Although this will trigger significant coughing, if the blood doesn't clear, this can be akin to drowning requiring emergent intubation and an attempt to isolate the bleeding.

We can use a device called a **double lumen endotracheal tube** and/or an **endobronchial blocker.** One branch of the tube is inserted into the part of the lung that's bleeding, and a special balloon catheter is placed into the airway. This isolates the bleeding part of the lung and helps the blood not to spill over to the parts of the lung that are still functioning.

d. Pleural Effusion:

Even without infection, cancer itself induces a significant amount of inflammation. This can attract a lot of extra liquid and cellular material that ends up accumulating outside the lung but inside the chest. This fluid pushes against the lungs and compresses them making it harder for you to breathe. This fluid is called a pleural effusion.

The pleural effusion can be further complicated if it gets infected and/or becomes bloody. Removing the fluid may require drainage with a needle (**thoracentesis**) and/or catheter through the chest called a **chest tube.** This rarely requires the ICU but can make you very sick when combined with other symptoms. See Appendix II C: Common Procedures in the ICU, for more tantalizing details.

iv. Cardiac Tumors

Tumors in the heart are rare and are often found incidentally. They are most often myxomas and sarcomas. They can cause obstruction of heart valves, interrupting normal blood flow causing heart failure and dropping your blood pressure. These may require support in the ICU in preparation for or recovery after surgery.

v. Colon, Rectal, Esophageal, and Stomach Cancers

Cancers of the gastrointestinal (GI) tract can cause significant complications that require ICU care. There are different sub-types of cancer common to the part of the GI tract from which they originate. They invade the wall of the gut with the most common complication being anemia from bleeding. This is usually a slow process, draining your blood over the course of weeks and months. If the amount of bleeding becomes more serious, symptoms include bloody diarrhea or vomit, and dangerously low blood pressure.

When a tumor causes an obstruction in the GI tract, everything starts to back up, causing severe pain, nausea, vomiting, and dehydration. If the obstruction gets bad enough to affect your blood pressure or cause severe electrolyte disturbance, then you may require the ICU. If this is treated surgically, you may also need the ICU post operatively to manage any surgical complications and assist recovery.

> ***ICU Confidential How Fast Did It Drop Edition:*** It's not uncommon for patients to present with very severe anemia and shockingly low levels of **hemoglobin**, the main protein in red blood cells that carries oxygen (4 or 5 mg/dl where above 12 is normal). You may feel tired and have modestly low blood pressure but otherwise feel okay. These are situations where you've been bleeding very slowly for a long time, so the body has had time to accommodate. You may still need the ICU if your anemia is very severe. On the other side of the scale, patients who come in profusely bleeding can have only slightly low hemoglobin levels because it hasn't had time to be diluted out. So don't let the hemoglobin itself fool you. Also, if you have anemia, get it checked out. It may not be a diagnosis in itself – you need to know what's causing it.

vi. Liver and Pancreatic Cancers

The most common primary liver cancer is hepatocellular carcinoma, responsible for about 75% of liver cancers. Cholangiocarcinoma is responsible for most of the rest. Major risk factors include alcohol use and hepatitis B, particularly after progressing to liver scarring (**cirrhosis**).

Complications from liver cancers that require ICU care usually result from liver failure or cirrhosis itself (see section F in this Chapter). Bleeding, confusion, and fluid retention are the main issues.

Another devastating diagnosis is **pancreatic cancer.** Because it is often advanced before it starts to show symptoms, it is frequently incurable at the time of diagnosis. We see you in the ICU as you run into complications from multiple chemotherapy attempts and/or after surgery, or from direct effects of the cancer. Too often with pancreatic cancer, we see you in the ICU because the cancer has metastasized, causing numerous complications like infection (**sepsis**), blood clots (**DVTs, PEs**), heart attacks, strokes, blockages in the bile duct, and uncontrollable pain.

> ***ICU Confidential Revolving Door Edition:*** We usually see you in the ICU when you are left without options for treating your advanced cancer. We also see you for acute complications after missing your medication, continuing to drink alcohol, or just because time has led to progression of your disease. We patch you up and get you healthy enough to leave, but you'll be back. Eventually, you come in and you don't leave (alive, that is, *everybody* leaves). There are supportive treatments for hepatitis, for helping you quit drinking, and the like. There are certainly treatments for liver cancer, including surgery and even liver transplantation if you're a candidate.

vii. Kidney and Other Urinary System Cancers

Common cancers of your urinary system include renal cell carcinoma, bladder cancers, and cancers of the urethra. During initial presentation and after treatment, the main complications include bleeding and urinary obstruction, as well as kidney failure, that can be severe enough to require management in the ICU.

viii. Breast, Ovarian, Cervical, and Testicular Cancers

This is a large group of cancers that can cause significant complications requiring ICU care. Common breast cancer concerns include pain control, and complications from surgery, radiation, and chemotherapy or immunotherapy.

Ovarian and cervical cancers can cause significant bleeding and swelling, including fluid accumulation in the abdomen. Testicular cancer can likewise cause significant swelling and pain.

While they are unlikely to be severe enough to cause an ICU admission, sepsis, blood clots and all the usual complications of cancer can be life threatening.

ix. Muscle and Bone Cancers

Sarcomas and primary bone cancers are rare but can cause significant localized and systemic complications. Cancers in the muscle and soft tissues can press on critical organs or blood vessels. Cancers of bone can also be very painful and lead to pathologic fractures including in the spine. This can lead to spinal cord compression, an emergency that may cause paralysis if not rapidly addressed. If very diffuse, bone cancers can also lead to dangerously high calcium levels requiring immediate therapy in the ICU.

x. Skin Cancer

Melanoma rarely leads to ICU admission itself except when widely metastatic and causing other regional and systemic effects. Other skin cancers, like basal cell and squamous cell, are very common and can be cared for in the dermatology office.

xi. Leukemia, Lymphomas, and Sickle Cell Disease

Acute leukemias can cause severely low red blood cell counts (anemia) and low platelets (**thrombocytopenia**), which can lead to uncontrolled bleeding. Leukemias can also result in severe immune deficiency through low white blood cells counts (**neutropenia**), or through having too many abnormal white blood cells that can't effectively fight infection but can clog blood vessels.

Cancer of the lymphatic system (**lymphoma**) can also be very dangerous, causing low blood counts and affecting your ability to fight infections.

Treating these types of cancers can lead to killing many of these abnormal cells all at once where the dead cells spill their contents into your blood. This leads to a complication called **tumor lysis syndrome** (**TLS**) which may lead to severe electrolyte disturbances. TLS can cause kidney failure, heart dysfunction, seizures, and even death. This can quickly become an emergency requiring rapid intervention and close ICU monitoring.

Although not cancer, another potentially severe blood disorder is **sickle cell disease**. It can cause very severe pain syndromes requiring sedation, as well as low blood oxygen and anemia since the red blood cells have a very abnormal shape. **Acute Chest Syndrome** can occur which causes severe chest pain and low oxygen levels requiring ICU care. Treatment typically consists of oxygen, pain control, fluids, and transfusions while providing supportive care.

xii. Metastatic Disease

As noted above, when cancer has spread beyond the place from which it originated, and has traveled through the bloodstream or lymphatic system, it is considered to be metastatic. Different types of cancers seem to prefer spreading to particular places in the body. For example, prostate cancer commonly spreads to the bone, while colorectal cancer commonly spreads to the liver and other abdominal structures.

Once someone has metastatic disease, it typically limits treatment to non-surgical options since it is felt that the cancer is already in the blood stream and this in part defines it at a higher (or more advanced) stage. There may still be a role for surgery to provide palliation but rarely cure."

ICU Confidential Catch 22 Edition: The adage "You have to be sick enough to get chemotherapy but healthy enough to survive it" leaves a very narrow treatment window when you're hospitalized. What happens when you are too sick because of the cancer to get the cancer treatment that will make the cancer better and you less sick? While there are some situations where chemotherapy can be started while you're in the ICU, the reality is that when you are in the ICU from complications of cancer like sepsis, heart attacks, blood clots, and strokes, chemo will only kill you faster and so you are stuck.

ICU Confidential Honesty is Invaluable Edition: When cancer becomes advanced, we can only hope that your oncologist has introduced the concept of **palliative care**, and that we are not the first ones to discuss things like **Code Status** and **Hospice** (please see Chapters 10 and 11). Unfortunately, all too often we in the ICU seem to be the first ones to tell you that your cancer is terminal. Granted, there is often a disconnect between what the oncologist tells you and what you hear since they are as guilty as we are in preferring the discussions to be optimistic rather than realistic. This ultimately does you a disservice as it robs you of the opportunity to prepare, of giving you the time to do what you need to do, see who you have to see, and prepare for the decline to come. It also deprives you of the chance to plan on where you want to die and how.

Not having these frank and honest conversations ahead of time often catches families off guard and may create distrust and skepticism about the severity of your condition. It may make you angry at the cancer, and that anger is naturally taken out on the messenger. We work very hard to engage your oncologist and communicate with one voice.

As hard as it is to hear, knowing the truth about where you are in the disease process is a gift you never wanted but shouldn't die without.

ICU Confidential What Makes You God Edition: Physicians are notoriously bad at making accurate prediction about when you will die. It's because we don't know. While we know the survival statistics in general, we don't know what *exactly* will happen to you as an individual. As such, we always try to be careful when we let you know how good or bad things are. We do tend to overestimate your odds the more we like you and the longer we know you (psychology 101).

There's also what I refer to as the ***Cone of Uncertainty:*** when you are healthy with a new cancer diagnosis, there's a wide range of timelines and possibilities. The sicker you are, however, the more accurate our predictions become. By the time you're in the ICU for your advanced cancer (on multiple pressors, requiring life support), we know what will happen, just not exactly how quickly.

J. Organ Transplantation

When organs are failing beyond recovery, organ transplantation may be an option. Some organs are more available, easier to replace, and and offer better survival once transplanted. Organ transplantation is rarely achievable in an emergency and almost always requires a long period of evaluation, follow-up, and extensive outpatient testing. This helps determine whether a candidate is physically, emotionally, and socially able to handle the rigors of getting a transplanted organ and the lifelong care that follows.

Organ transplantation is an exceedingly complicated topic and what follows are very brief descriptions of the most common transplants we see in the ICU.

i. Kidney

When kidneys fail, we can replace their function with dialysis. This can sometimes be done at home while you sleep (**peritoneal dialysis**), or at special centers that circulate your blood out of your body and "clean" it before returning it to you (**hemodialysis**). While this technology is lifesaving, it still makes your life more difficult, and shorter. More kidneys are transplanted annually in the US than all other organs combined. This has become a much more routine operation, and patients usually tolerate the surgery without having to go to the ICU unless there is a serious complication.

ii. Liver

Liver transplantation is one of the more complicated types of transplantation. This is partly because patients with liver failure are typically much sicker (no "liver dialysis" exists to support them). This is also because the liver is a larger and more surgically complex organ to transplant, much more prone to bleeding, bile duct issues, and graft failure. Bleeding, confusion, and infections are the most serious complications. Prolonged ICU stays before and after the transplant are not uncommon.

iii. Heart

Now you're really in the big leagues. Uncontrolled heart failure's last chance is a whole new heart. This is a very complicated procedure requiring life support, **ECMO**, and a whole slew of advanced interventions. Very skilled transplantation programs with advanced surgical and critical care expertise are required.

iv. Lung

Lung transplantation is similarly complex and requires highly specialized resources to perform successfully. Organ rejection, infection, surgical complications, and respiratory failure may require prolonged ICU stays. If you are an overachiever, and both the heart and lungs are failing together, you may need a combined heart and lung transplant, adding a whole other dimension of complexity.

v. Bone Marrow

There are certain blood cancers and blood disorders of the bone marrow where you may need an infusion of new bone marrow. Your diseased bone marrow must be eradicated first using chemotherapy and radiation. This is not surgery but carries significant risks like organ rejection and infection. Severe sepsis and bleeding are the typical complications that may require the ICU.

vi. Pancreas and Intestine

These transplants are much rarer and require significant expertise and support in the ICU. Complications from the often extensive surgeries as well as from graft failure can be severe and require a whole team of experts to manage.

vii. Brain (just kidding)

As much as you feel you may need one, it's not available (yet). Maybe take a vacation.

> ***ICU Confidential:*** Organ transplantation remains perhaps the most resource intensive therapy that medicine can offer. There are not enough organs to go around, and there are many ethical considerations. From a justice perspective, the cost of a single liver transplant can pay for nutrition, vaccinations, and preventive health care for a classroom of kindergarteners, for a year. On the other hand, if your child suffers from heart failure and needs a transplant, you will move heaven and earth to save them.
>
> Because of the intense amount of resources, organ transplant remains a privilege and is strictly and objectively controlled based on who has the best chance of survival, and what everyone else is giving up. Remember, someone typically has to suffer a profound tragedy to give the organ (living donors also undergo significant risk). And, if the organ goes to someone that doesn't survive, another person on the transplant list may die waiting for that organ. Organ transplantation is nothing short of a medical miracle but is challenging on many levels.

K. Multi-Organ Failure or *All of the Above*

Failure of a specific organ can lead to a domino effect of all the body systems shutting down. The body depends on everything working together, so when a major organ starts to struggle, it pulls everything down with it. Say you have a heart problem that drops your blood pressure (heart failure). This damages your kidneys (renal failure) and liver (liver failure). This leads to fluid accumulation in the lungs (respiratory failure). This eventually leads to severe confusion and even coma (brain failure). It's like the middle to end of the end.

L. A Shout Out to the Fluffy Among Us

Being significantly overweight is not a medical condition that in itself requires the ICU. It may, however, have significant consequences for your medical care in general, and in the ICU specifically. Your anatomy may make procedures, including placement of large IVs (**central lines**) and **intubations**, more technically difficult and more prone to complications. It may be harder to physically turn you in the bed or mobilize you after surgery, leading to more skin breakdown and ulcers on your backside.

Morbidly obese patients also may be at higher risk for malnutrition because the protein levels plumet during critical illness, even though you are technically overweight. It may be more difficult to do other basic things like getting you transported for testing. You may also be denied certain interventions such as organ transplant because obesity affects survival. On the other hand, there's evolving data that suggests you can do as well as lower weight individuals such as in **ECMO** outcomes during COVID.

> ***ICU Confidential Fluff Daddy Edition:*** There are many stereotypes that lead to medical bias against overweight individuals. It's so pervasive that many healthcare systems require sensitivity training to counter this. In taking care of obese patients, we have to realize that it's much more complicated than not having the willpower to eat less. There are many factors at play, both hormonal and psychological. As health care providers, we work very hard to counter this bias and recognizing it is the first step. On your end, own it. Let us know that you understand you're very overweight, you recognize how it may be affecting your health, and that you're really trying to correct this. Let us know that you'll help us take care of you every way you can, and that you deserve the same quality care as anybody else. I've never met a caregiver that is able to maintain their bias when a patient owns this.

ICU Confidential Big, Beautiful, and Fit Edition: The risk for medical problems generally increases with weight, including heart disease, strokes, diabetes, high blood pressure, sleep apnea, even certain cancers like breast and colon. There is more evidence, however, that it is actually the level of fitness that's most predictive. We call this the **anaerobic threshold**, or the limit of activity your body can endure before it switches how it gets its energy where lactic acid level gets too high. The more conditioned you are, the higher this threshold. That's why cardio type exercise is so important for risk reduction, although weight training also has a role. Fitness levels are hard to measure (think giving blood samples while running on a treadmill hooked up to wires and a mask). We use weight as a proxy for fitness because 1) it's easy to measure, and 2) it often correlates to fitness. In reality, if you have a fit "overweight" person who can run a 10-minute mile and keep going, and an out of shape "skinny" person who can't jog to the end of the block, that overweight person may carry lower risk of complications. So, work on fitness first and the scale will follow.

8 Life Support in the ICU

There are specific interventions so essential to your survival in the ICU that they deserve their own chapter. Rather than describing a specific medical diagnosis, this section focuses on the main life support interventions encountered in the ICU: the **ventilator**, lifesaving interventions for low blood pressure (**shock**), **advanced cardiac support** therapies, and **extra-corporeal membrane oxygenation** (**ECMO**), the ultimate life support/replacement technology.

While these therapies can be started in the ED (or on the hospital ward in response to a **Code Blue**), it's in the ICU where they are usually performed and maintained. Other technologies like dialysis and feeding tubes are also considered forms of life support, but they can be done outside the ICU and are described elsewhere (such as in Chapter 7: Medical Journeys by Diagnosis).

A. Respiratory Failure and Being on a Ventilator:

When you can't breathe well enough to keep up with the oxygen and carbon dioxide demands of your body, you have **respiratory failure.** If the condition causes a low oxygen level, we call this **hypoxemic** respiratory failure. When it causes an increase in carbon dioxide, we call it **hypercarbic** respiratory failure. We further delineate it as **acute** or **chronic**, or acute on chronic (you can't breathe well in general, but now it's even worse).

Numerous conditions can lead to respiratory failure, including pneumonia, congestive heart failure, lung collapse, neurologic muscle disease, and losing the ability to protect your airway, such as during a stroke, coma, or drug overdose.

As we manage and treat the underlying problem, we can support your breathing to keep you alive, including through artificial means. We do this through a series of steps, starting with supplementing your oxygen through a nasal cannula. This can only do so much, and we then switch you to an oxygen mask and, if that's not enough, we initiate a special **high-flow oxygen** delivery system. If you still need extra help, we may use a forced air mask that is similar to an external ventilator called **non-invasive ventilation**.

If this is still not enough to safely support your breathing, we proceed with **intubation** and place you on a ventilator. This section describes what a ventilator does, what you experience, and the process of coming off once your breathing improves. For more information on specific oxygen therapies, see Index I: Machines and Things. For an exciting description of how we intubate you, see Appendix II: Common Procedures in the ICU.

i. What Is a Ventilator:

A **ventilator** is a complex type of air compressor. It mixes purified air with varying amounts of **oxygen (O_2)** and pushes it through a tube which is connected to your lungs. Using air pressure, it forces air into your lungs with every breath.

When you are ready to exhale, it drops the pressure to passively let you breathe out. Connecting the ventilator to your airway is a tube called an **endotracheal tube**, or **ETT**. It goes down your throat, through your vocal cords and into your windpipe, also known as the **trachea**. If you've had a tracheostomy, a special version of the tube goes into your trachea directly through your neck.

A ventilator allows us to control the amount of air that is delivered with every breath, how much force is being used to deliver the breath, how much oxygen is in that air, how often the breath comes, and whether you trigger the breath or if it's given automatically (and that's just the start). There are different sets of ventilator parameters we call ventilator modes, and your specific situation determines how all these settings are managed.

Ventilator Function	Translation
Frequency or Rate (breaths per minute)	How many breathes per minute the ventilator delivers
Tidal Volume (ml)	How much air is given with each breath
Fi02 (%) [Fraction of inhaled oxygen]	How much oxygen is in the air that the ventilator delivers
Inspiratory Pressure (mmHg)	How much force the ventilator gives with each breath
Positive End-Expiratory Pressure (PEEP)	How much force is provided by the ventilator when you are breathing out
Trigger	How each breath is triggered – either by patient effort or automatically (or a combination).

ii. Why You May Need a Ventilator:

As described above, the first reason to need a ventilator is because your oxygen levels are too low despite the use of non-invasive methods. Delivering oxygen directly to the lungs is what the ventilator does best.

The next reason to be on a ventilator is if the **carbon dioxide (CO_2)** levels in your blood are too high. This means that you are not breathing deeply enough or often enough to get rid of the carbon dioxide your body generates. The ventilator takes over the work of breathing when you are too weak to breathe on your own, or if your respiratory muscles are failing for other reasons. The ventilator will bring relief and provide a mechanical way to get rid of the CO_2.

Intubations are also used for **airway protection**. When you've lost the ability to keep things out of your lungs because you are very confused (**obtunded** or in a **coma**), such as after a stroke or drug overdose, or are at high risk of vomiting because you have a severe stomach bleed or colonic obstruction, then you may need a ventilator to protect your airway and keep you from choking to death.

iii. How a Ventilator is Initiated

If intubation is planned and we have time to prepare, the process is smoother and safer. We get all the right equipment at the bedside, have the proper personnel gowned and ready, have the right sedatives drawn up, and have time to discuss the procedure with you and family to get your informed consent. This is the best-case scenario for you and for us — it's a much calmer and controlled experience with a lower risk of complications.

More often, placing a patient on a ventilator is an emergency. In this scenario, you are undergoing a rapid decompensation or a **Code Blue** situation, and chances are you are dying or already dead (and turning "blue"). You may be losing or have already lost consciousness or are just struggling to breathe. Preparation is limited in these circumstances, and everything happens as quickly as possible. There is a greater risk of complications, including failed intubations. For a more detailed description of the procedure, take a deep breath and check out Appendix II: Common Procedures in the ICU.

> ***ICU Confidential Early Warning System Edition:*** You don't want to be on a ventilator. We don't want to put you on one, either. We would only do so if the alternative was worse (death through suffocation). When we run into situations where your goals of care are consistent with life support, but you are declining intubation until "the last minute," this creates a more dangerous situation and that last minute can become your actual last minute. When we recommend intubation pre-emptively, it's because we see it coming, so please listen. On the other hand, when you refuse our medical advice and things go badly, it releases us from liability. This gives us ~~no~~ a little comfort.

iv. How a Ventilator Supports You

Delivering oxygenated air directly into the lungs under force is the most effective way to help the lungs do what they do, which is exchanging oxygen for carbon dioxide. This serves two functions: One, it provides the oxygen needed for your cells and therefore your organs to function and keep you alive. And two, by getting rid of carbon dioxide it maintains the acid-base balance in the body needed to sustain life. When all else fails, the ventilator allows the best way to do this by maximizing what function your lungs are still able to provide.

A ventilator and the endotracheal tube it's attached to also provides a direct highway into the lungs. This highway is protected from the mouth, throat, and esophagus (which connects the back of your throat to the stomach). As such, it prevents food, mucus, and other materials from going into the lungs and causing additional damage. In situations where you can't protect your airway, being on a ventilator does it for you.

v. You're On a Ventilator, Now What?

Now we've bought some time. While we support you on a ventilator, we control your oxygenation (O_2) and ventilation (CO_2). We try to optimize the ventilator settings to deliver the most benefit with the least amount of harm. We check your vital signs, labs, including **arterial blood gas** results, oxygen levels as reported by the continuous **pulse oximetry**, respiratory patterns, x-rays, and feedback from the ventilator itself. We use all this data to monitor how well the ventilator is supporting you and adjust the settings on an on-going basis.

Being on a ventilator can be very difficult. You cannot talk, you cannot eat, you cannot get up to move your bowels, and it is typically very physically and mentally uncomfortable. Because your mobility is very restricted, you start to lose muscle mass almost right away, and the chance of bed sores, skin breakdown and infections starts to increase.

You are hopefully appropriately sedated throughout the process. We aim for the minimum amount of sedation needed to keep you comfortable so as to minimize the side effects of the sedatives, including low blood pressure, low heart rate, and lasting effects on your mental status.

We can and do wake you up, especially when we feel you are ready to come off the ventilator (see the next section), and when checking your neurologic status. This is called a **sedation vacation** or **spontaneous awakening trial (SAT)**. During those times when your sedation is low enough, you may be able to communicate with gestures (careful, now), point to a picture of a word or activity on a picture card ("pain" or "bathroom"), or sometimes even write. We also use this break from sedation to see if you can start breathing on your own while on the ventilator, a process called a **spontaneous breathing trial (SBT)**.

The physical force from the ventilator can further damage the lungs if the pressure settings needed to keep you alive are too high, which can cause **acute respiratory distress syndrome**, or **ARDS** (see Chapter 7: Medical Journeys by Diagnosis), lung collapse, and ventilator associated pneumonias. Make no mistake, this is a very uncomfortable intervention physically and mentally. But for all its negatives, it is a machine that keeps you alive with the goal of giving you time to heal from whatever made you need a ventilator in the first place.

ICU Confidential, Talk to Me Edition: Even when you are seemingly awake while on a ventilator, it is often difficult to tell exactly what you understand and your capacity to make decisions. You can be awake enough to make eye contact and follow simple commands (like "squeeze my hand") but are very limited in how much you understand. Sometimes we can give you a pen and clipboard with the intention of having you write out what you want us to know. It takes time and patience to try and understand you, so make sure we don't rush the process while we are rounding. We can at least leave a medical student behind (and we do).

vi. Coming off a Ventilator (Liberation)

Coming off a ventilator in the ICU is different from coming off a ventilator after a routine surgery. In the surgery scenario, you could hopefully breathe well before the surgery, so all you have to do is wake up from the anesthesia to breathe well after surgery. This usually takes only a few minutes after the anesthesia is turned off and you take control of your own breathing.

Coming off the ventilator in the ICU happens more slowly and through a step-by-step approach. The first thing that must happen is that whatever got you on a ventilator in the first place must be improving. For example, once your pneumonia is effectively under control and your oxygen requirements have come down, or your congestive heart failure is improved with diuretics, or your confusion is behind you, you are ready to start weaning from the ventilator.

Coming off the ventilator requires your participation. We take you on a sedation vacation where we turn off the IV piña colada (sedation) and allow you to wake up as completely as possible. We then set the ventilator to hand over more of the work of breathing to you until you are essentially breathing on your own with minimal help from the ventilator. We optimally need you to be fully awake and participating, doing most of the breathing using your own strength, and requiring a reasonable amount of oxygen support.

After an appropriate duration of breathing through the ventilator using your own strength (typically 30-60 minutes), the **respiratory therapist** (**RT**) puts you through what are called **weaning parameters** to see if you've got the right stuff. For example, we measure how much air you can take in when you take as deep a breath as possible and check the force you can generate when you exhale as vigorously as possible. This is all done through the endotracheal tube and monitored through the ventilator.

When your mechanical lung parameters look good, the RT performs a final deep suction, deflates the endotracheal tube's balloon cuff to release it from your trachea (making sure air is going around it, called a **cuff leak test**), takes off the duct tape/holder keeping it in place around your mouth, and finally removes the endotracheal tube. This is called **extubation**, or *liberation* from the ventilator.

To help your transition to breathing fully on your own, sometimes we extubate you to a nasal cannula with extra oxygen flowing through it, and sometimes you need the external mask that delivers support with air pressure through a BPAP machine (Appendix I: Machines and Things).

We check to see if you are ready to come off the ventilator every day, sometimes several times a day. With an illness that improves rapidly, you may need a ventilator only for a few days. With more prolonged illness, this can take many days or even weeks of working hard every day, trying to increase your level of independent breathing little by little.

We can take ventilator weaning as slowly as you can tolerate, making small victories every day. If things are not going well, and the original problem isn't amenable to being solved, or additional complications happen, you get stuck on the ventilator. We keep trying, but if the situation persists, additional decisions will be required. None are good, but hope is not lost. When you are ready, see Chapter 10: Code Definitions and More, and Chapter 11: What Happens After the ICU.

ICU Confidential 5 Star Edition: Spontaneous awakening trials (SATs) partnered with spontaneous breathing trials (SBTs) where we test your ability to get off the ventilator every day are a major quality marker for ICUs. When done correctly, patients come off ventilators faster, leave the ICU sooner, and have a greater chance of surviving through hospital discharge. Most high-quality ICUs have protocols that are driven by the ICU nurse and respiratory therapist to wake every patient and see if they can breathe on their own every day. If we don't check if you are ready to come off, we can't know. You do have to be medically stable enough where the stress of trying isn't dangerous, but it applies to everyone else. Don't be shy about asking if your loved one had an SAT and SBT today!

ICU Confidential What's the Big Deal Edition: When we think about *life support* we often consider the ventilator our main intervention. It's often the line in the sand used to define when your time has come, so much so that it gets its own code status designation ("Do Not Intubate"). On the one hand, it's just another procedure we use to support you through your medical journey. On the other hand, it's such a significant intervention that can take so much from you. If we can't get you off the ventilator, it becomes your life going forward. As we discuss here and in Chapter 10, going on and staying on a ventilator is a very personal decision, and we try our best to give you enough time and information so you can make the right choice for yourself.

B. Hemodynamic Failure, Shock and Pressor Management

Blood pressure is maintained by several factors – how well your heart is working, the tone of your blood vessels, and if you have enough blood/volume in circulation. Think of your circulatory system as a large network of pipes delivering freshly oxygenated blood to the tissues of your body. It drops off the oxygen, nutrients, and other raw materials to the tissues and picks up carbon dioxide and the byproducts of metabolism (waste). Blood with low oxygen and high carbon dioxide is pumped through the lungs where oxygen is replenished, and carbon dioxide is dropped off to be exhaled. The cycle starts again when oxygen is delivered throughout the body and used in the formation of cellular energy so all our tissues and organs can function correctly.

Oxygen-rich blood is pumped through the kidneys where excess fluid and byproducts are removed to be turned into urine and eventually urinated. Oxygen-rich blood is pumped through the muscles to keep us moving and breathing, the liver to remove toxins and add important chemicals, and the pancreas to pick up insulin and chemicals to digest food.

Most importantly, blood is pumped through the brain where oxygen is used in the process of creating energy to keep those neurons firing.

The forces and pressure that drive this blood flow can be referred to as **hemodynamics**. When this system is in jeopardy, we call this **hemodynamic failure** which leads to **shock**. Shock describes a loss of blood pressure that compromises blood delivery to (and from) our organs, causing them to suffocate and quickly lose function. We use different interventions to correct this, including IV fluids and special medications called **pressors**.

i. The Mechanics of Blood Pressure

It can help to think of our circulation as a pressurized system of pipes. A pump moves the fluid through pipes in a closed system, getting it to different locations where it gets filtered or where additives are infused, and recirculates it. In your body, the heart is the pump, the blood vessels are the pipes, the blood is the fluid, and the different organs are the locations the fluid must be pumped through.

The blood vessels that carry blood away from the heart are called **arteries**. They have muscles in their walls so they can constrict and relax, providing local variability of blood flow. This allows them to direct more blood to vital organs when the total system pressure drops. Arteries can also open and expand near the skin to drop your body temperature when you are getting too hot (or embarrassed). They can also prioritize flow in response to activity, like the muscles, heart, and the lungs when exercising, the digestive track when you're eating, and the brain when you're reading this book.

The main artery carrying blood from the left side of the heart (left **ventricle**) is your **aorta**. Your aorta branches into smaller arteries that head off to different regions of your body. The arteries get smaller as they divide, until they are like a tiny single pipe leading to your kitchen faucet. At this point they are called **capillaries**, and they are small enough to exist within all of your tissues numbering in the billions.

Blood has many different cells that act as containers floating in fluid (**plasma**), and it is in your capillaries that the drop off of oxygen, sugars, and lots of other chemicals needed for your tissues to function correctly occurs. In exchange, carbon dioxide and cellular waste products get loaded into the blood cells and plasma to be carried away.

Capillaries merge with other capillaries and become larger blood vessels eventually joining one of two very large veins returning blood to the right side of the heart (the **superior vena cava** collecting blood flow from our upper body, and the **inferior vena cava** collecting blood flow from the lower body). The blood is then pumped through the lungs and returned to the left side of the heart ready to repeat the circulation cycle.

The vessels that return blood to the heart are called **veins** and compared to arteries they are much less muscular and are designed to carry blood at a lower pressure. They have one-way valves to prevent backflow.

When these mechanisms are overwhelmed and the system loses pressure, that forward flow can't continue as efficiently, your blood pressure drops, and a cascade of bad things starts to happen. As noted above, this is called shock.

> ***ICU Confidential Math Nerd Edition:*** Blood pressure in the ICU is calculated as the mean arterial pressure (**MAP**), the average pressure in your arteries during one complete heart cycle. The generally accepted limit under which the MAP is considered too low is 65 mmHg. The calculation takes the **systolic** blood pressure (the high number obtained at the end of a cardiac contraction) and adds two times the **diastolic** blood pressure (the low number obtained at the end of heart relaxation) and then divides this by 3 ((SBP + 2*DBP)/3).
>
> For a "model" blood pressure of 120/80, this would be (120 + (2 x 80))/3 = 93; notice it is much higher than the lower limit of 65. When it is lower than 65 mmHg, there is danger of not getting enough blood to your vital organs, so we intervene to help increase your blood pressure.

> ***ICU Confidential I Run Low/High Edition:*** Although 65 mmHg is a good rule of thumb for the minimal blood pressure to effectively circulate blood throughout the body, some people live at lower pressures, and some people are used to higher pressures. We take this into account when correcting your blood pressure. The actual blood pressure goal is whatever it takes to avoid organ damage by delivering enough blood flow (not too high, not too low) for your organs to function normally.

ii. Why Blood Pressure Drops

Your body can go into shock for a number of reasons. You may experience major trauma, say your arm just got torn off by a Sasquatch and blood is rapidly escaping from your body due to the torn blood vessels / burst pipes (this is called **hemorrhagic shock**). If you become severely dehydrated from not drinking enough fluids or from peeing too much you may have **hypovolemic shock**.

It can also be more complex, like when your body has an overwhelming infection which causes a dysregulation of your immune system where it goes out of control. This affects your heart and your blood vessel tone and permeability, leading to pump failure and leaky pipes, or **septic shock** (also called **distributive shock**).

If you suffer a heart attack or arrhythmia and your heart is damaged, then you can go into **cardiogenic shock** (pump is broken). If you have a large blood clot in your lung circulation (pulmonary embolus) that leads to acute right sided heart failure, this is called **obstructive shock** (pipe is blocked).

A common example of temporary shock is when your nervous system is briefly dysregulated, like losing arterial tone from a fright or by bearing down too hard (**vasovagal response**). You usually recover quickly and don't need the ICU.

iii. Why Shock Is Dangerous

Your body can endure low blood pressure only for short periods of time. Without an adequate blood supply delivering oxygen and essential chemicals, your organs start to suffocate, and irreversible damage can occur. The heart especially needs a steady blood supply to keep its muscles fibers working. Without this constant blood flow, the heart starts to fail, which sends your body into a rapid cycle of decline.

A whole slew of inflammatory chemicals like adrenalin are released in your body to counteract low blood pressure as tissues start to suffocate. This leads to an increase of lactic acid, and the body starts to fail metabolically. When the brain doesn't get enough blood flow and/or the blood is too acidic, you get confused and eventually pass out. If not corrected, death ensues.

iv. How We Fix It

While we work to identify and correct whatever led to your shock in the first place, it is essential that we immediately support blood flow to the vital organs. We give you **intravenous (IV)** fluids (and blood products if you are bleeding), and when these are not enough, we reach for special medications, only given in emergencies, and in the ICU.

By rapidly infusing IV fluids and blood products as appropriate we increase the pressure by (over)filling the expanding/leaking pipes that are your blood vessels. This is called **fluid resuscitation** and is the mainstay of surviving sepsis and other shock states. If you are in septic shock we would infuse 30 ml/kg of fluid in the first several hours. For example, if you weigh 200 lbs, that's just under 3 liters of fluid. If you are bleeding, a **rapid infusion protocol** is initiated where IV fluids and blood products can be mechanically infused.

When fluid resuscitation is not enough to raise your blood pressure, we start special IV medications that put the heart into overdrive, increase blood vessel tone, or both. This artificially increases your systemic blood pressure and directs blood towards your essential organs. The medications that do this are called **vasopressors (or pressors)**.

Think of pressors as different versions of adrenaline, the hormone or neurotransmitter that triggers your main fight or flight response. There are 5 common pressors in practice: norepinephrine, vasopressin, epinephrine, phenylephrine, and dopamine. They have their differences and can be applied in combination when needed (see Appendix III: Medications in the ICU).

If shock is caused by **heart failure**, we add mechanical support in the form of advanced heart therapies including specialized medications and mechanical pumps (see section C coming up, and Appendix I: Machines and Things).

v. How Pressors Are Titrated

As the blood pressure goes down, the dose of pressors is increased to try to compensate. The ICU nurse has a titration protocol of what pressor to use, and how much to adjust the dosing, all based on your mean arterial blood pressure. We also have protocols for when to add a second or third pressor and how they can work together.

When things improve and the blood pressure goes up, the number and dose of pressors goes down. This is generally a very good sign. Your medical team manages the order and initial dosing of pressors.

vi. Complications From Therapies

Going into shock is life-threatening, and treating shock requires complex decisions and close monitoring. If we infuse too much fluid into your veins and your heart can't take it, this fluid can saturate your lungs and interfere with breathing (**pulmonary edema**). Too much fluid can also result in upsetting your body chemistry, creating severe electrolyte imbalance.

Pressors also have a slew of side effects. They strain your heart and blood vessels pushing them to work harder which can lead to

arrhythmias, heart attacks, and **ischemic** digits (tips of fingers and toes turn black). The higher the dose and the more pressors you need, the greater the danger.

Pressors also require an IV infusion, usually into a large vein using a **central line catheter**. Using a central line is especially important if you require high doses of pressors for an extended period of time as they can harm smaller blood vessels and cause severe tissue injury. Placing and maintaining this type of catheter has its own hazards (see Appendix II: Common Procedures In the ICU).

> ***ICU Confidential Between a Pressor and a Hard Place Edition:*** Pressors are generally considered a type of life support. If you are maxing out 3 pressors and your blood pressure is still low, this is a very ominous sign as the likelihood of passing away is high. Pressors may (should) be included in the conversation about **Code Status** (see Chapter 10: Code Status Definitions and More).

C. Advanced Cardiac Support:

You may have had a series of heart attacks, or you are lucky in love but unlucky in genetics and have dilated **cardiomyopathy** (heart muscle failure) or **amyloid** heart or one of a number of other disorders that affect your heart function. You may be on some powerful medications chronically, but your heart is still struggling. Now is when you need advanced support for your heart, and this is managed in the ICU.

i. How We Evaluate Your Heart Function

Our first step is figuring out what kind of support your heart needs. This requires initial testing including an ultrasound of the heart **(echocardiogram, or echo)**, an EKG, and some laboratory tests. An echo is packed with information about your general heart function, how well your heart valves open and close, and more. If the echocardiogram or EKG results concern us, we may proceed to **cardiac catheterization** where we evaluate your coronary arteries for blockages, and your cardiac pressures using a special catheter going through your blood vessels.

Another special catheter called a **Swan Ganz** or **Pulmonary Artery Catheter (SGC, PAC)** may be left in the blood vessels extending through the right side of the heart into the pulmonary (lung) artery. This will be used to guide therapy as it gives direct pressure and other measurements including from direct blood samples that help us know what specific types of assistance your heart requires (See Appendix II: Common Procedures in the ICU).

ii. What is Advanced Cardiac Support

Special interventions aimed at improving heart function or mechanically supporting circulation with a pump or procedure fall under the category of advanced cardiac support. These interventions are generally divided into medications and medical devices, and a combination of these may be required. This may be temporary such as when your heart needs time to recover from a heart attack, or longer-term as a bridge to heart transplant. Sometimes, versions of these interventions can be used more chronically (as **destination therapy**) at home.

a. Medications

IV medications that improve how well the heart beats may be required to safely maintain your hemodynamics. This includes medications like **milrinone** and **dobutamine**. They initially require careful titration and need central line access in the ICU, as well as frequent monitoring through a special catheter inserted into the blood vessels feeding your lungs (pulmonary artery or Swan-Ganz catheter). These medications are different from pressors as they specifically target heart function. They can also be transitioned to chronic use. If you are already on one of these medications at home and come into the hospital for an unrelated problem, you don't necessarily need the ICU. More on specific medications in Appendix III: Medications in the ICU.

b. Devices

Mechanical devices designed to directly assist the heart include a special mini pump that sits just outside the heart in the aorta, the large artery leaving the heart. Called an **intra-aortic balloon pump (IABP)**, this device inflates when the heart relaxes, thereby giving an extra *push* of blood. This helps feed blood to the coronary arteries as well as to the rest of the body.

A special heart pump that is continuously working to move blood forward can be inserted directly into the left side of the heart.

This is called a mini left ventricular assist device (for example, an **Impella**®)and it comes in different sizes and strengths. These and other similar mechanical interventions require on-going monitoring, adjustment, and troubleshooting which means needing to be in the ICU. Check out Appendix 1: Machines and Things for more information.

If you've suffered a cardiac arrest, another ICU intervention is a special protocol called **targeted temperature management (TTM)**. Also known as **therapeutic hypothermia**, this process intentionally drops your core body temperature to help improve your neurological function. Although not technically there to support the heart, it is used to protect the brain when the heart has acutely failed. TTM requires deep sedation and special equipment, and can lead to arrhythmias and other complications, so it should only be performed in the ICU.

ICU Confidential Now What Edition: When you are being sustained on one of these advanced medications and/or mechanical devices, the reason is to give your heart time to recover from whatever insult it suffered, or to give us time to actively fix the problem (such as surgically correcting a failing heart valve or coronary artery blockage). In the case of severe and irreversible heart damage, you may require a heart transplant. If you are not a candidate for a transplant, some of these advanced therapies may be transitioned to chronic use, including at home. This requires a lot of help and support and is what we call destination or palliative therapy. Some of these interventions, especially the mechanical ones, cannot be done at home. Before proceeding to one of these interventions, you must have an exit strategy including if you are willing to live with these devices for weeks or months in the ICU.

D. Extracorporeal Membrane Oxygenation (ECMO):

We've discussed ways to help the breathing (ventilator) and the heart (advanced heart therapies). But what if that isn't enough to support these organs? What if you needed to completely replace their function? The machine that does this is **Extra-Corporeal Membrane Oxygenation**, or **ECMO** for short.

ECMO has its origins in coronary bypass and other open-heart surgeries where the heart must temporarily be stopped while being operated on, and blood flow has to be diverted to a circuit outside the body, artificially oxygenated while having carbon dioxide removed, and pumped back into the body. ECMO is complex, takes significant expertise to operate, and is fraught with technical and ethical considerations. ECMO is more than life support, it is *life replacement.*

ECMO definitely requires the ICU, and what follows is a brief description of why. Run, don't walk, to Appendix II: Common Procedures In the ICU, for more details on how ECMO is performed, and Chapter 10: Code Status Definitions and Difficult Decisions.

i. Types of ECMO

Depending on whether only the lung function requires replacement, or if it is the heart that is struggling, two main types of ECMO exist:

a. Venovenous (VV) ECMO

When your lungs are no longer able to oxygenate and ventilate, even with full support from the ventilator, ECMO is your ultimate option. A very large catheter is inserted into a central vein such as the **femoral** vein in the groin or the **jugular** vein in the neck. This catheter carries blood out of your body to the ECMO machine. In ECMO, your blood is pumped through a membrane device that infuses it with oxygen while removing carbon dioxide; this essentially serves as an artificial lung.

Your blood is warmed back to body temperature, gets a blood thinner additive to prevent it from clotting in the ECMO circuit, and is pumped back into the venous circulation using another large catheter that has been placed downstream of the first one. (Sometimes the two catheters are combined into one with the return port positioned beyond the collection port.) VV-ECMO replaces the functions of the lungs as the returned blood is already artificially oxygenated and depleted of carbon dioxide.

The most common conditions that may require VV ECMO include severe pneumonia that turns into **acute respiratory distress syndrome (ARDS)**, or other severe inflammation and scarring in the lungs. The high levels of oxygen and air pressure needed from the ventilator may not be enough to raise your oxygen levels sufficiently. What's more is that these high levels of ventilator support can add to inflammation resulting in further lung damage.

ECMO allows the ventilator to be set to minimal settings so the lungs can "rest" and have time to recover from whatever assaulted them in the first place. Sometimes ECMO is a bridge to a lung transplant when lung recovery is not possible.

b. Veno-Arterial (VA) ECMO

When your heart has given out and isn't able to support your circulation despite all our attempts including advanced cardiac interventions, or you have a combination of heart and lung failure, then VA-ECMO can be used to temporarily replace the functions of both the lung and heart.

In VA-ECMO, the blood is taken out of the venous circulation like in VV-ECMO, but it is returned directly into the arterial side of the circulation thereby bypassing the heart as well as the lungs. The VA-ECMO pump is set high enough to support systemic blood pressure thereby replacing the pumping function of the failing heart. The oxygen is added to and carbon dioxide is removed from the blood, just like in VV-ECMO, so the function of the lungs is also replaced. You may no longer have a pulse or a 2-tiered blood pressure, just a constantly pressurized blood return.

VA-ECMO is performed not only in the operating room while undergoing heart surgery, but sometimes during recovery if the heart still isn't working well and needs more time to regain function. VA-ECMO is also provided when heart failure occurs after a severe heart attack or inflammatory process that affects the heart muscles. If the heart failure is not reversible, VA ECMO is often the last step before a heart transplant.

ii. Complications and Contraindications

ECMO carries high risks of complications, such as bleeding (including in the brain), infection, blood vessel rupture, kidney failure, and more. If there is a mechanical failure of the ECMO circuit (the pump, the tubing connections, the oxygenator), or if the catheters get dislodged or become clotted, the results can be catastrophic. Infection can develop along the catheters where they enter the skin, or in the blood stream, leading to sepsis. The longer you're on ECMO the greater the possibility of complications.

ECMO has been used for much longer and with much greater success in the pediatric population. Kids appear to be much more resilient and can tolerate this therapy with better success, including when very young.

Outcomes in adults have undoubtedly improved over time but are still not as good as they are in kids. For adults, the best success is in the military where young, otherwise very fit and healthy soldiers experienced severe trauma or infection and developed ARDS. Their survival rates with ECMO are significantly better than the general population.

When VV-ECMO is applied to older and sicker patients, most notably during respiratory infection pandemics (H1N1 influenza, COVID-19), the outcomes strongly favor younger patients who are otherwise healthy (55 years old or younger, no other organ failure, and in reasonably good medical condition prior to the event). Outside these scenarios, most patients died anyway.

ECMO is also a very resource intensive therapy, requiring lots of special equipment and personnel. On the one hand, it gives people a final chance at life. For some, however, it only prolongs the inevitable, so very special attention must be given when deciding who to offer this therapy to.

> ***ICU Confidential Death Panel ECMO Edition:*** Only more advanced and comprehensive medical centers offer ECMO at present. Most of these centers will have a committee that reviews all ECMO proposals outside generally approved protocols. During times of extreme stress on the medical system (like during the COVID pandemic of 2020+), committees typically comprised of a cardiothoracic surgeon (they put in the catheters), ICU specialist (they manage the ECMO), and organ specific specialist (a cardiologist or pulmonologist, or both) would decide who would benefit most from this technology. The hospital's ethics committee is also typically involved. The case is presented, the panel deliberates and then comes to an agreement. Similar to decisions made by an organ transplantation committee that considers which patients would best benefit and are most likely to survive, these ECMO life-or-death decisions aren't left to a single individual.

iii. Day to Day Management, and Tomorrow Management

In addition to a very experienced and qualified ICU nurse taking care of only you, there is an ECMO technician (**perfusionist**) that oversees the minute-to-minute functions of the ECMO circuit, and an experienced intensivist physician to oversee the care. A cardiothoracic surgeon is also available to fix any catheter site issues.

While there may not need to be changes very often, they are all there to troubleshoot and quickly correct any potential disruptions as these can be deadly. As noted above, blood clots, bleeding, catheter malfunction or dislodgement, problems with the pump assembly, the warmer, the medication infusion circuit, and more can occur. A back-up ECMO circuit needs to be available at a moment's notice.

Adjustments to ECMO are made in gradual steps based on **arterial blood gas (ABG)** analysis. An ABG shows oxygen and carbon dioxide concentrations in the blood and allows the perfusionist to optimize how much and what type of help the ECMO circuit is providing. Daily chest X rays confirm that the catheters are where they should be. Blood pressure readings from arterial lines help the physician adjust how forcefully the circuit is made to work. Labs done throughout the day further guide these changes.

If you've been on ECMO for a while, changes to your ECMO settings become less frequent. If you are in the heat of the moment, adjustments continue to be made until you are stably unstable.

> ***ICU Confidential Walk This Way Edition:*** You are typically sedated and immobile while on ECMO. In the pictures you see of patients "walking" with ECMO, there are usually about 15 people to help them and the patients themselves are usually young and otherwise healthy (think teenager waiting for a heart transplant). While you can be kept alive for a long time with ECMO, most agree that you don't live with ECMO. ECMO should not be initiated if there is no exit strategy or little chance of overall survival.

iv. Weaning Off and De-ECMOing

When your lung and heart function improves and you need progressively less help from the ECMO circuit, we begin to wean you from ECMO. This is balanced with the ventilator, as well as with how much support your heart may be needing from specialized medications. Once the ECMO settings have been providing minimal support for some time, ECMO can actually be placed on stand-by prior to removing the catheters. If you continue to show improvement, all breathing and heart functions are fully transferred to you, and the catheters can be removed. This transition can take days or weeks depending on your age, overall health, and what condition(s) led to you needing ECMO in the first place.

ECMO is offered only as a *bridge* to something else. Like many things in the ICU, it's meant to give the body (in this case, the lungs and/or heart) time to recover, or time to get a replacement through organ transplantation. The risks must be justified, and only patients who are otherwise in fairly good shape survive, so that's who is offered this therapy.

This brings us to the other way to get off ECMO. When there is no other side to the bridge, or when the cost of continuing to search for one is no longer acceptable to you, compassionate withdrawal of ECMO can be offered. Like withdrawal of any life support technology, this is ethically and legally the same as not starting ECMO in the first place. In practice, however, it's much harder for you and your family to physically stop something that is keeping you alive. More on this and other uplifting conversations in Chapter 10: Code Status Definitions and More.

v. ECMO During Code Blue or ECPR

One notable application of ECMO is providing it during active resuscitation (**CPR/ACLS**) in a **code blue**. In an attempt at resuscitating you if your heart has stopped and you have stopped breathing (see Chapter 10: Code Status Definitions and Difficult Decisions for more details), you can be emergently placed on ECMO if you meet very specific criteria. This is called ECPR.

Because of the resources that must be immediately available (surgeon to place the catheters, the ECMO machine with a back-up, the perfusionist to run the ECMO machine) this is only available in very select centers. The criteria for those who will benefit remain the same as ECMO outside a code blue situation – young, otherwise healthy patients with potentially reversible disease.

ECPR is an emergent treatment option that will likely become safer and more mainstream as the technology develops and experience builds.

9 Medical Ethics and the ICU

Medical ethics are general rules of behavior based on what is considered right and wrong in the practice of medicine. These aren't necessarily specific to the ICU, but they do get tested there more than in other medical arenas given the serious medical conditions of ICU patients.

As the next several chapters deal with significant end-of-life issues, I feel that it's important to first label and define the elements that form the foundation for how we, as physicians, approach difficult decisions in your care. The following is a brief description of the guiding principles of medical ethics with a hint of ICU flavor.

A. Beneficence

The principle of beneficence dictates that your physician acts in your best interests. This means that the physician puts your needs before those of the hospital, themselves, and even other patients (see *Justice* below). In other words, your physician should always be working on your behalf.

This seems simple but "best interests" can be difficult to define. The medical scenarios in the ICU often make patients and physicians choose the lesser of two evils. When a procedure that can cause harm through complications is balanced against the risk of not performing this procedure and risking death, the concept of "best interests" gets cloudy.

End-of-life decisions make this even harder. For example, is putting you on life support where you will remain for weeks and months before dying but will honor your wish to stay alive longer in your best interest? Or is it in your best interest for us to make sure that when you pass away it is with comfort and not hooked up to machines even if that means dying sooner?

These are always very personal decisions influenced by your life experience, spiritual beliefs, family inputs, and much more. Our job as physicians is to work on your behalf by providing all the information we have, offering guidance based on our knowledge and your goals, and ultimately supporting your choices as best as we can.

B. Non-maleficence

Non-maleficence is the "do no harm" tenet that your physician swears to uphold when reciting the Hippocratic Oath during medical graduation (even though we technically swear it to the god Apollo). This means that we as physicians should never purposefully do anything with the intent of harming you.

The concept of non-maleficence struggles with the same difficulties as beneficence. For example, we may feel it is harmful to submit a patient to CPR in the context of an end-stage terminal illness, but you may feel it is harmful to let your family member pass away if there is even a very small chance of extending life.

It's also important to distinguish situations where pain or discomfort may be part of your treatment. If a life-saving procedure causes pain, we are still ethically acting with non-maleficence since the intent of this procedure is to save your life (see the concept of double effect below).

C. Autonomy or Self-determination

Autonomy is the right of competent adults to make informed decisions about their health care. This wasn't always standard practice. Decades ago, physicians decided what was right without input from the patient, often letting the patient know only after they had already performed a surgery or procedure.

Autonomy is a right fought for through a number of landmark court cases giving the right to decide to the patient. This right to self-determination doesn't give you the right to ask for anything you want but gives you agency to guide your medical care.

The concept of autonomy creates shared decision making where we provide you with the medical facts and our opinions of the benefits and pitfalls of the available options, and *you* ultimately get to choose what the right decision is. Importantly, this means you can also *decline* interventions.

D. Informed Consent

The concept that you as the patient should be informed of the benefits, complications, and alternatives of any medical treatments recommended by your health care team prior to agreeing to them is called informed consent. Informed consent for procedures and surgeries is documented in a standardized manner that requires your signature or witnessed verbal agreement. This should include a comprehensive description of the procedure, why the procedure is recommended, and what the alternatives are.

Informed consent should also include a discussion of potential complications and be free of coercion or bias. That doesn't mean we can't share what we as physicians think is the right option for each situation and why. What we shouldn't be doing is pushing you into a decision you may not be ready for.

> ***ICU Confidential Emergency Edition:*** If a medical emergency is unfolding where we do not have the luxury of time, we are obligated to do what we feel is medically necessary in that situation. This typically applies to situations where you may be unconscious or unable to give consent and we can't reach your medical proxy, or you are actively dying in front of us. In the US, **Good Samaritan laws** ensure that a provider who renders treatment in good faith in an emergency is not held liable for lack of consent.

> ***ICU Confidential Just Sign Here Edition:*** It is not uncommon for the nurse to hand you a consent paper (or electronic signature pad) and direct you to sign without further explanation. This should absolutely not be happening, and you should insist on getting all the information you need before consenting to a procedure. Fully explaining the procedure protects the clinician as much as it does the patient. After all, if there is an expected complication, having an informed consent allows us say that you agreed to the procedure with full understanding of the risks involved.

E. Justice

There are several layers to the definition of justice in the context of medical ethics. First is the idea that we should treat all patients equally and equitably, with every patient getting the very best available care options. Justice also means that limited resources should be distributed in a way that benefits the most people in the most meaningful way. These two ideas may contradict each other: if we offer a few people very costly interventions, we will have to eventually deny other people even basic therapies because resources are limited.

For example, the field of organ transplantation is trying to provide individual justice by offering a life-saving organ in an objective way based on your likelihood of long-term survival and irrespective of your ethnic or professional status in life (you still must have medical insurance and social support). On the other hand, the enormous resources needed to save one person with an organ transplant arguably take funds and expertise away from basic medical needs that can potentially save many more people.

Your physician is generally obligated to put your needs first, and those of the greater patient population or even the whole of society second.

F. Confidentiality

Confidentiality in the doctor/patient relationship is considered ethically and legally protected. This means that a physician cannot disclose a patient's private health information to a third party without the patient's consent. This helps build trust between patient and physician and encourages honesty. The exception is intent to harm yourself or others, suspected child abuse, or in certain public health concerns like communicable diseases (tuberculosis or HIV, for examples).

In the ICU, this can create friction as you may not want to reveal your health conditions like cancer, HIV/AIDS, or other STIs to your family (they are not directly affected in this scenario), and so they may not have the whole picture if they have to make decisions on your behalf. This explains why if you become incapacitated, your health care proxy is obligated to receive this information and may decide to share it with others.

G. Double Effect/Double Intent

The idea that you are doing something good even if this action can have other negative consequences describes the concept of double effect. This can be applied to causing pain during a procedure because the intent of the procedure is to make your underlying condition better. Likewise, this applies to giving strong pain medications to alleviate your suffering at the end of life, even though it may lead to you dying sooner. This is considered ethical (and legal) because the intent is to provide comfort, and you are ultimately passing away from your disease, not from the pain medications (not to be confused with euthanasia, see Chapter 10: Code Status Definitions and Difficult Decisions).

H. Ethics Consultation

There are circumstances in the ICU when there is significant disagreement between you, your family/healthcare proxy, and the medical team. Common scenarios include disagreements about end-of-life care, who is appointed as the decision maker if you are incapacitated, and determining situations of medical futility.

There may be financial conflicts of interest where if you die, your family stops getting your social security check (or gets an insurance payout). There may be conflicts of interest between what you designated in your living will and what your medical power of attorney wants because of their religious beliefs that may be different from yours.

For these scenarios and more, most medical centers have a designated team of professionals consisting of ethicists, social workers, and physicians who are external to your case and are tasked with applying legal and ethical principles to help guide you, your family, and your medical providers. Your physician may ask this team to see you to provide an ethics consultation. They will interview you, your family, and the medical team to provide an outside expert opinion.

An ethics consultation can be essential in helping bridge the gap in understanding between all the people involved in your care. It will also provide an independent audit of your situation in the context of what is considered legal and ethical.

ICU Confidential Ethically Speaking Edition: The purpose of the ethics consultation is to lay out the facts and dispel the emotional cloud that sometimes distorts these facts. This may help you focus on what's important to you and your loved ones. While they usually have no direct legal or medical authority, their official recommendations can be used in legal or administrative actions.

I. A Case Study in Ethics: Justice and the Cost of Healthcare

Uncle Jack drank his liver to near death. He quit 6 months ago but now his liver is completely failing, and he'll die without a transplant. That transplant will cost the health care system about a million dollars (in 2025), and that's just the initial hospital encounter. The immunosuppressant drugs, the constant testing and surveillance and complications are all extra, not to mention the risk of relapse. But if he gets a new liver, there's a 75% chance he'll still be alive in 5 years. He can spend time with his family, have a good quality of life, and perhaps support others in their recovery.

Great Aunt Alois has advanced dementia, and her food goes into her lungs when she eats or produces saliva. She is 85 years old. She is generally confused but still has periods where she recognizes your voice, and there is a special connection when she squeezes your hand that shows part of her is still with you. Keeping her on life support and a feeding tube and subsequently caring for her in a chronic ventilator facility will cost about $500,000 dollars per year, not including the inevitable complications that lead to more procedures and hospitalizations.

The cost of public-school lunch is about $4. The cost of immunizing a child through their entire childhood is about $600, divided over 18 years. The cost of 8 months of prenatal care (without insurance) is about $2000. And that's just in the US – it's significantly cheaper in the developing world.

If Uncle Jack is allowed to pass away from his liver disease, the resources saved can provide prenatal care for about 500 expectant mothers, *saving the lives of about 3 babies*, and giving many more a healthier start in life. If Great Aunt Alois goes to hospice where she slips into a coma and passes away in a month or so, the resources saved can *feed and shelter about 300 homeless kids in the US, for a year* (or about 4,000 or more children in most parts of the developing world, for a year).

Would it be ethical to include (or exclude) this information in the informed consent? Would it be right to treat an individual with beneficence if that would mean you couldn't do the same for the next patient? Is denying a potentially lifesaving intervention the same as maleficence? Should the right to self-determination have limits, and who gets to decide these limits? Easy questions to have over coffee; talk amongst yourselves.

Of course, the above scenarios assume this is a zero-sum situation - that the resources saved from a transplant or a chronic ventilator facility will be directly used to provide prenatal care or feed hungry children, and we all understand how complicated that gets. You may argue that we should be doing both. You may also argue that taxes and healthcare spending are already too high. These are difficult decisions to say the least, and we as physicians have to focus on our individual patient; the larger questions that address population systems and policies are left to public health experts, administrators, and (*sigh*) politicians.

10 Code Status Definitions and Difficult Decisions

Dying is the only 100% guarantee in life, which makes appropriate planning important even when you are in good health. The question, of course, is not if but when (and how). In the ICU, thinking about the future is especially important since the risk of dying is especially high.

There are several key medical concepts to know and understand when it comes to planning for medical emergencies and decisions regarding end of life. This chapter reviews topics like code status, advanced directives, and the specific interventions surrounding death itself. These are among the most important things you can learn about, and plan for.

A. Historical Perspectives – CPR, Defibrillators, and Ventilators

Before the advent of scientifically driven technological intervention, there wasn't much one could do once you were actively dying or have already died (where the heart and breathing have stopped). The decision was basically to call your particular theological representative and hope you're right about the afterlife.

With the recognition that some blood circulation can be maintained through chest compressions there came an intervention we could do in an emergency. This was previously called closed chest massage, and eventually evolved into what we now call **CPR** or **cardiopulmonary resuscitation.**

When the heart stops or is no longer beating in a way that moves blood through the circulation, such as in an arrhythmia, you no longer have a pulse. If this is not immediately corrected, all the organs start to quickly die.

CPR can keep the blood circulating to the vital organs because as you push down on the chest you increase the internal pressure and push the blood forward through the arteries and veins. Because the valves in the blood vessels allow blood to flow only in one direction, in the short-term CPR gets the job done. Think about pushing your car while in gear. You can't get very far this way, but you may be able to get the engine started.

To perform CPR correctly the provider must push on the chest at about 100 compressions per minute, at a depth of about 2 inches, while the patient is lying on their back. Compressions have to be forceful to work, and this is why ribs often get broken.

For CPR to be effective, it must also be started right away. It only buys you a little time to try to reverse or correct the injury that caused the heart to stop beating in the first place. This can mean shocking the heart with electricity (**defibrillation**), or administering an **anti-arrhythmic** medication, or getting you breathing again by clearing a choking airway or expelling water from the lungs after drowning. Even outside the hospital, CPR absolutely saves lives, and *everyone* should be trained in how to provide it correctly.

The next major advance in resuscitation care came with the recognition that shocking the heart with electricity can reverse a specific deadly arrhythmia called **ventricular fibrillation**. A ventricular fibrillation cardiac arrest can happen during a heart attack but could also happen for other reasons, or even spontaneously.

Appropriately named, **defibrillators** eventually became commonplace and can now be seen hanging in public areas, malls, and many other commercial spaces – almost every place with a first aid kit. Defibrillators have visual and audible instructions, analyze and automatically provide a shock once activated, and can save a life in those crucial minutes ahead of when emergency medical help can arrive.

The next element of acute life support, **artificial ventilation**, started with humble beginnings of mouth-to-mouth breathing (resuscitation). This was performed alongside CPR as rescue breathing. With the advent of special oxygen masks and more readily available microchip-based ventilators, the 1960s and 1970s saw **intubation** and mechanical ventilation incorporated as part of the emergency response.

Interventions used to stabilize and resuscitate patients were eventually protocolized. First, **Basic Life Support** (**BLS**), which included things like CPR, rescue breathing, and defibrillation, was established, followed by **Advanced Cardiovascular Life Support** (**ACLS**), which included guidelines for medications and for emergently placing patients on ventilators.

As CPR, defibrillation, and mechanical ventilation became widely adopted, the standard of care expected them to be automatically applied in every possible case of death. Eventually (circa the 1990s), physicians and patients recognized that there were very clear situations where these interventions were inappropriate and even went against the wishes of the patient. These were situations where there was no chance of recovery, like in cases of injury incompatible with survival or in terminal illness. There was also the formal recognition that patients should have the final say in what happens to them at the end of their lives.

As the rights of patients to refuse certain treatments became recognized, this created a cultural practice shift to patient **self-determination** (also referred to as patient **autonomy**), won through a number of major court decisions. This principle established that patients (and their families) would be able to decide what they would or would not want to go through when they died.

> ***ICU Confidential It Gets Worse Edition:*** Before the transition from "everyone gets CPR" to "patients always get to decide" there was what can be referred to as the "slow code" scenario. The slow code referred to physicians deciding who gets the aggressive all-out effort and who gets a resuscitation attempt in name only. There were even cases when charts would have a label (like a purple sticker) to indicate such a status. Analysis of this practice revealed a bias towards patients with no insurance or of certain ethnicities (translation: poor and non-white individuals). This practice slowly went away with cultural enlightenment (and likely some law suits). Today, records are very strictly maintained, including careful and independent documentation of the resuscitation attempt itself, including what medications were given and when, and if all the right steps were followed.

B. BLS and ACLS

Basic Live Support (BLS) and Advanced Cardiovascular Life Support (ACLS) are a set of protocols that govern what your health care team does in a medical emergency such as cardiac arrest. It codifies the above interventions such as when and how to perform CPR, how to apply a defibrillator, and when to consider intubation.

BLS focuses on recognition that there is a problem ("Are you okay?"), checking for a pulse, starting CPR, and applying a defibrillator. It gives the provider step-by-step instructions for when to initiate these steps and how to correctly perform them.

ACLS builds on BLS by introducing specific medications and more advanced interventions. These protocols define what steps are taken in a code blue situation (see below) and also apply to different arrhythmias. It specifically teaches providers how to recognize life threatening arrhythmias and what medication and procedures to use to save the patient's life.

BLS and ACLS are established by the American Heart Association® with broad input and standardization and are intermittently updated with the latest data. Your medical providers are certified in BLS and ACLS through standardized training that is periodically updated and repeated.

C. Code Blue

Code blue is the ubiquitous code name used for a set of protocols designed to try to resuscitate someone who is dead or actively dying, such as when their heart stops or goes into a deadly arrhythmia, or when spontaneous breathing comes to a stop. This is in the overhead hospital announcement that makes our heart skip a beat as well. The code blue activates a dedicated medical team that comes rushing in with specialized medications and equipment (just like you see on TV, quickly but somehow also in slow motion).

A **crash cart** with emergency medications and a **defibrillator** is quickly wheeled into the patient's room. Nurses start connecting **EKG** wires, drawing up medications, and checking IV access. A respiratory therapist is getting an **Ambu bag** to forcefully deliver oxygen and an **airway box** with **intubation** equipment. Doctors are helping where needed with emergency procedures like obtaining large IV access and **intubation**. One of the physicians is the medical team leader, giving the orders and directing the effort.

Chest compressions (**CPR**) are started right away. Large doses of **epinephrine** and other drugs to jump-start your circulation are also given. If your heart is in the specific arrhythmia that can be shocked back to normal (**ventricular fibrillation**), electric shock is delivered through pads placed on the chest and back, called **defibrillation** (handheld paddles are no longer used). When required, a tube is placed down your throat and into the windpipe to deliver oxygen and artificial breaths directly to your lungs with a **ventilator**.

While these first steps are taken to keep you alive, the medical team will be trying to figure out what caused your code so they can hopefully fix the underlying problem. We are examining you, and reviewing your labs, X-rays, EKGs, and medical record, and giving emergency medications to reverse possible causes.

Each round of CPR is 2 minutes long, at which time we very briefly stop to check your pulse and heart rhythm, and administer medications and/or shock. We are also trying to get in touch with your medical proxy to let them know what is happening, and to get additional guidance as to your wishes.

The code blue continues either until you are stabilized or until after anywhere from 15 to 30 minutes or longer when the team runs out of interventions and there is agreement that nothing more can be done. At this point, we consider "appropriateness of continued resuscitation" as the team leader asks if anyone has any additional ideas or objections, and we stop.

If this happens to you outside the hospital, the immediate survival rate is unfortunately about **10%**. In the hospital, the immediate survival rate is about **25%**, with under **10%** of patients surviving to hospital discharge

ICU Confidential Not as Seen on TV Edition: Code blue is very traumatic in nature. Ribs get broken, electricity jolts the body, and ventilator tubes are inserted into sometimes hard to access airways. On television, code blue is portrayed as a typically successful attempt at reviving you with full recovery in a matter of minutes. The patient seems to wake right up, high fives the nurse, and gets ready to be discharged home. In truth, even when successful, the resuscitation process only buys you time to reverse whatever caused you to code in the first place. The longer the attempt at resuscitation, the more likely you are to have brain damage from lack of oxygen and organ failure from lack of circulation. If you do survive, the shape you're in depends on many factors, but will not be better than before whatever caused you to code in the first place.

> ***ICU Confidential Case by Case Edition:*** When the case is truly beyond recovery, but the family hasn't yet come to terms with what has happened, we proceed with code blue at the same maximal intensity, but we don't take it out to 30+ minutes, as at this point the code is being performed for the family, not the patient. When the patient is young, the code is unexpected, and/or we feel the underlying catastrophe is recoverable (heart attack or arrhythmia in a younger person – yes; major stroke in an end-stage cancer patient – no), we keep the resuscitation going and even consider truly extraordinary measures when they are available (see upcoming section on **ECPR**).

D. Code Status Topics and Definitions: GOC/Full/DNR/DNI/CMO

Above, we described the general steps taken during a code blue. You as a patient have a choice in deciding what happens to you in such medical emergencies. Here we'll provide some definitions of terms defining these options, from having the medical team perform extraordinary measures to try to bring you back and keep you alive, to letting nature take its course.

Goals of Care (**GOC**) is the general term we use to define end-of-life conversations. They refer to anything having to do with overall health goals towards the end of your life but specifically address the degree of medical interventions that would be acceptable to you under the circumstances. You may reasonably ask why anyone's goals would be different than "My goal is to be healthy and live forever." The caveat is that the goals must be reasonably achievable and applicable to your situation. And, of course, this is never simple.

For example, "I want to live as long as I absolutely can no matter what." Does that mean on life support? Does that mean unable to talk or independently use the toilet or recognize your loved ones? Does that mean being completely unconscious, or worse, fully aware but **locked in** where you can't move, and no one realizes you are fully aware? Would a balance be acceptable? For example, if you are paralyzed on a ventilator but can communicate with your eyes by pointing at individual letters on a speech-generating device (think Stephen Hawking), would that be acceptable?

These are very individualized choices with almost unlimited permutations. I think the most important thing is to ask yourself what is most important to you. In the US and much of the medically well-resourced world, these are choices dictated by the individual.

Interestingly, most laws are enshrined giving patients the right to refuse treatment (not the right to demand treatment). In other parts of the world, the physician makes the call, taking your wishes into account but placing the emphasis on the actual medical situation. In places where resources are just not available, these choices are made for you.

When we meet you and are ready to have this conversation, we first gauge your knowledge of what goals of care are, and if you've already had a chance to think about these issues. We have this discussion in the context of a living will if there is one (see the upcoming section on advanced directives). We then proceed to define code status options.

I begin the conversation by emphasizing how important it is to first understand these terms, and try to reassure patients that this conversation happens with every patient admitted to the hospital, including the ICU. I note that while we don't expect medical emergencies to happen, we must prepare for them by knowing your wishes so we can respect them if the time ever comes. The following is a transcript of how I describe code status to patients.

i. Full Code

When someone enters the hospital, we offer every medical, technological, and other intervention that is appropriate to their care. This includes testing, medications, procedures, surgery, and more, to help fix the underlying problem. Under **full code**, if you get so sick that your heart stops, or you stop breathing and are actively dying, we initiate chest compressions, otherwise known as **CPR**, shock the heart with electricity if appropriate, and place you on life support with a **ventilator** to try to bring you back. We cannot know ahead of time if we are going to be successful, or what state you may be in if we are able to bring you back. Full code is the default designation unless you tell us otherwise.

ii. DNR/DNI

In the second scenario, we do all of the above – the testing, treatment, technology, procedures and so forth, but if you pass away, or are getting so sick that you are unable to breathe on your own, we do not put you on a ventilator, or have you undergo chest compressions, or electric shock; we recognize that your time has come and let you go as comfortably as possible as you previously designated. This is called *allowing a natural death* and is what we refer to as **Do Not Attempt Resuscitation**, and **Do Not Attempt Intubation** or **DNR/DNI.** (In many facilities, DNR includes DNI, and we typically discuss them as part of the same order.)

Activating code blue and putting you through an attempt at resuscitation including initiating life support is completely appropriate when we just need extra time to fix an underlying problem. DNI/DNR, on the other hand, is appropriate when what made you so sick is *not* reversible or the price of trying to reverse it is unacceptable to you. In this scenario, putting you through these extraordinary measures in the context of a terminal illness in its final stages is not likely to get you back and may only prolong the inevitable in a very uncomfortable and invasive way.

We as medical professionals put DNR and DNI together in general. If you are actively dying from a respiratory arrest, it doesn't make sense to perform **CPR** without supporting your breathing by providing an airway, meaning **intubation** (DNI not DNR). If you are dying from a cardiac arrest, it wouldn't make sense to intubate you but not perform CPR or **defibrillation** (DNR not DNI). However, there may be very specific circumstances where differentiating DNI and DNR makes sense according to your philosophy or medical situation, and we consider these on a case-by-case basis.

> ***ICU Confidential Choose Your Own Adventure Edition:*** In some situations, we do separate the DNR and DNI as the intubation may be a line you would not want to cross while CPR and defibrillation may be acceptable. This may be applicable if you are at high risk for a reversible arrhythmia where you would be okay to get defibrillated, but you would not want to go on any other type of on-going life support.

iii. CMO (Comfort Measures Only):

When the medical problem becomes unfixable, or the cost of continuing to try to fix it is not acceptable to you, we can transition to focusing exclusively on your comfort. **Comfort Measures Only** is the designation we use for this scenario. We treat every symptom as completely as possible, including pain, anxiety, constipation

– whatever affects your quality of life at that moment. No more X-rays, blood draws, invasive procedures, or other interventions that don't directly contribute to your comfort.

If death isn't imminent, we usually upgrade you from the busy environment of the ICU to a calm and private room, or even a dedicated facility or home with support services. This is often understood as **hospice**. Hospice is actually a set of medical resources consistent with CMO, but one can think of it similarly. (We'll discuss this in Chapter 11: What Happens After the ICU.)

iv. Applying the Living Will

When we discuss code status, we always incorporate information from the living will if one exists (this is your advanced directive for end-of-life care; see section F for more on this). For example, if the living will specifies no desire for life prolonging measures and you are dying from terminal cancer, we clarify that the living will is consistent with Do Not Attempt Resuscitation and even Comfort Measures Only.

If you are incapacitated, after explaining definitions with your health care proxy, I share that we as physicians have only a small window in the life of your loved one and can never know them the way you do. I would tell your proxy that the responsibility falls to them to express what their loved one would want in this situation: "Imagine your loved one standing here and listening to our conversation. What would they say?"

I end the explanation part of the discussion by acknowledging how difficult these goals of care decisions are and emphasize that the family is not making the decision for you but only informing us what you as the patient would have wanted. (Of course, if you can speak for yourself, the conversation is with you.) We do encourage you to include family at the bedside both for your support, and for their understanding of your wishes by hearing them directly from you.

After discussing the definitions of code status and the different options, I will ask if you or your family have any questions. After clarifying any details and confirming your understanding, I will listen for your decisions and help guide you as to how we can help carry out those decisions. I never press for an answer to your code status – I never want to leave you feeling pressured or rushed and would prefer for you to think about these choices and discuss this further with your loved one. If time is very limited because you are already that sick, I will make sure you know this as well.

v. No Escalation of Care

When we talk about removing treatments already in place, it often creates an emotional burden on families since they are "taking something away." Even though legally and ethically it is considered the same as not starting it in the first place, removing care can have very different optics ("unplugging" grandma is emotionally not the same as not "plugging her in" in the first place).

A compromise to this is determining that while we do not take away anything already in place, we at the same time agree not to add anything else. This often applies to situations like escalation of **pressor** dosing (powerful IV medications that keep the blood pressure up), and additional procedures and interventions, along with not putting someone through a code situation (DNI/DNR). This is often more emotionally acceptable as you are still treating and giving time for the patient to recover, but you are not putting them through more interventions should they get even sicker.

> ***ICU Confidential Throwback Edition:*** In the past, having a DNR was akin to not being aggressive with your care. It wasn't quite like transitioning to hospice but was perceived as somehow not caring as much. I can tell you emphatically that this is no longer true (or legal), and that we are sometimes more aggressive or overdo certain therapies because we don't have the luxury of life support and ACLS should you die. Unfortunately, this idea that DNR equals less care had infiltrated the caregiver culture (nurses, physicians) and eventually to patient perception. It has been decades since this was true, but that stigma persists, especially among some older (thankfully) retired caregivers who haven't practiced for a long time. On the other hand, if you get even a whiff of this, make sure to correct your nurse or caregiver immediately.

vi. Code Status and Surgery

You may be in a situation where you've elected to be DNR/DNI, but that there is a procedure or surgery that aligns with your goals of care and would be acceptable to you. The surgery may be for pain relief or other forms of palliation but may require intubation for anesthesia. You can put a hold on, or rescind, the DNR/DNI designation for 24 hours or more to make it possible to have the surgery. You can also designate that if there is a major complication, or if you are not able to come off the ventilator, we transition to comfort care and/or compassionately remove life support if recovery is not expected.

ICU Confidential Exemption of Surgery Edition: Surgeons have to meet many quality markers, and one of the most important is the mortality rate, or how many patients survive for at least 30 days after surgery. This can create a situation where you are dying and surgery can help alleviate some suffering in the time you have left, but the surgeon is reluctant to operate based on how it will affect their statistics.

For example, I cared for an end stage cancer patient who underwent amputation of a finger that had ulcerated due to metastatic cancer going to the bone. Their life expectancy was only weeks, but amputating this cancer-ravaged finger provided significant relief and allowed the patient to be present with their family rather than overly sedated from pain medications. This surgeon did the right thing ethically, morally, and in every other way, even though it may have blemished their otherwise excellent mortality rate statistics. If a surgery or procedure can provide significant palliation, it may still be reasonable even if you've got a very limited life expectancy, and you can make this point with your physician.

vii. Patient Autonomy and Physician Input

Patient autonomy is paramount to a successful health care culture. This should not mean that we expect you to have all our expertise and experience, no matter how well we explain the situation to you. We as physicians have the responsibility to give our best opinion as to what you should do. We do this by taking into account your medical situation and putting it together with who you are as a person, and, most importantly, what your goals are. We do this by channeling our many years of experience and study. We do this by listening to you.

ICU Confidential Killing the Messenger Edition: Please don't get upset at us for discussing your prognosis in realistic terms. I typically tell you when I first meet you that I will always be completely honest about how good or bad things are. If you don't know the whole truth, you cannot make fully informed decisions. When it comes time and your prognosis becomes clearer, I will talk to you about resuscitation, about compassionate withdrawal of technological support, and about hospice. I make sure you know what we know, and what we don't.

This is not because we are giving up or don't want you to get better. It's because at that point, the battle has changed from fighting the unwinnable battle against the cancer, or heart failure or stroke, to fighting a winnable battle for a dignified, and peaceful death.

Unless you tell us otherwise, the futile attempt at resuscitation will be terrible and traumatic, and legally mandated. This remains a leading cause of burnout for your ICU nurses and physicians – the futility of what we consider tantamount to torture instead of offering you comfort in the last moments of your life.

E. Making the Decision

Your medical team takes many factors into considerations when helping you decide on whether and how to continue care. This includes many details of your medical conditions, your health and functional capacity prior to coming to the ICU, and the degree of reversibility of your current situation. It can be helpful to understand how we look at these factors.

i. Prognostication

The ability to predict what will happen to you is termed prognostication. To give you the best prediction about your medical outcomes, we use data from medical studies that look at what happens to people in your situation and are also guided by our professional experience. There's been a lot of study on this topic as our advice relies on our ability to prognosticate well. If we are 100% sure you are going to die a prolonged and painful death, we would be giving different advice than if we were only 20% sure.

To help you understand your options, we can bring statistics into our conversation. If we follow a thousand people like you that went through what you are going through, and, say, 5% survived but were dependent on life support, we can tell you this and may recommend hospice. While that helps you with planning, it doesn't predict with certainty that you will be among the 95% of people who don't survive, or the 5% that do. The thing about statistics is that if it happens to you, it's 100%, and if it doesn't, it's 0%. Statistics also can't tell you if this will happen in an hour or a day or a week.

We often also give predictions based on survival rates. This is common in cancer based on how advanced your disease process is. We call this cancer *staging*, and we often quote the 5-year survival rate based on what stage your cancer is in. Remember, these are average numbers. Some patients will survive longer, while some will die sooner.

The closer you are to death the better we are at predicting it. If you are on your 5th chemotherapy regimen and your cancer is progressing and you've already coded twice and are on multiple pressors because of overwhelming sepsis, you are going to die. We are right every time on this one. If you come in because of a heart attack and we open the artery and you are otherwise healthy, we are right almost all the time that you will be okay (for now).

> ***ICU Confidential Are We Friends Edition:*** It may surprise you to learn that physicians are humans, with human biases. It has been demonstrated that the better we like you, the more overly optimistic we tend to be in our predictions, perhaps because we want that to be the right prediction. This is more so in the clinic setting where we get to know you over the years, but the consequences also make their way into the ICU. Due to these good intentions, we often provide a more optimistic picture than is realistic for your situation. We are also more reluctant to give you bad news because we don't want to disappoint you. A good doctor, however, will be aware of this bias, and will tell it to you straight, no matter how much it hurts you (and them), because without honest information, you end up losing precious time, and you may be consenting to interventions you would otherwise avoid.

> ***ICU Confidential AI Edition:*** As the world of artificial intelligence infiltrates all aspects of technology, medicine is not being left behind. As I write this, the research volume of AI generated programs that predict medical outcomes including in the ICU is quickly growing. By the time you read this, we may be quoting an AI generated prognosis score that can predict your ICU survival better than we ever could before. It will still be a matter of statistics, however, and until AI can predict your medical future at 100.0%, there will always be some uncertainty.

ii. Best Case/Worst Case

A good way to consider your options is to think of best- and worst-case scenarios. What follows is a version of a standard example used to teach clinicians:

Say you come into the hospital with bowel obstruction. You have a history of inflammatory bowel disease, you've had multiple operations, and you live in a nursing home because of an extensive array of other medical problems including heart failure and the consequences of a prior stroke. You are at high risk for anesthesia and complications from surgery. The surgeon discusses surgery to alleviate your obstruction versus focusing exclusively on comfort through palliative care with hospice (for a more detailed discussion of palliative and end-of-life care, see Chapter 11: What Happens After the ICU).

In the best-case surgery scenario, you have the surgery and recover in the ICU over a period of 4 to 5 days. You will be on a ventilator after the surgery and with some luck you can come off in a few days and can be transferred to a regular hospital room. You can eventually start eating and stool will exit into a colostomy bag. The several weeks in a hospital bed will further decondition you, leaving you with a long road to recovery, which would be defined as your life in the nursing home prior to the bowel obstruction. With some luck, you can work hard to gain the necessary strength in a long-term acute care hospital or rehabilitation facility before returning to the nursing home. You'll never be quite as good as you were before the bowel obstruction.

In the worst-case scenario, you have a surgical complication in the operating room, you suffer another stroke in the ICU and you can't come off the ventilator. You are maintained in the ICU for over a month with ventilator-associated pneumonia and your surgical wound gets infected. You die on life support in the hospital, or (perhaps worse) you are transitioned to a chronic ventilator facility and are kept alive on machines where you cannot talk or eat or get out of bed. You wait for the next medical complication when you ultimately pass away.

Your surgeon will give you an idea of how likely the worst versus best case scenario will be for your specific situation. Given this, the option of management with palliative care will also be introduced. In this option, you do not proceed with surgery and are given medications to alleviate any pain or discomfort. You will have time with your family at your bedside. There is a small chance that the bowel obstruction will spontaneously resolve, but it is much more likely that you will die from this. If you do, it will be on your terms where you will be comfortable and in as natural a state as possible.

These scenarios may help you evaluate your choices. Your surgeon should give you the opportunity to share what is important to you. Using this information, they should be able to share their opinion of what you should do that best aligns with your goals and values.

ICU Confidential Not a Menu Edition: Going to your doctor should not be like going to a drive through at McDonald's®. Your physician should present you with the information you need to understand the situation and inform you of the possible outcomes from the available options. They should elicit what your goals and wishes are and *recommend which option fits those goals best.* Your physician should never impose on your right to decide, but they shouldn't stand passively by without giving you their best advice.

When your physician hesitates, it may be because they don't know what the best option would be, and they should discuss that openly with you. Physicians shouldn't hesitate because they don't want to take on that responsibility; they don't have that luxury. If your physician is silent, *ask*!

On the flip side, I am surprised how often the patient or their family do *not* ask their physician for advice when it comes to end of life care. They ask friends and relatives with no medical training and no knowledge about the patient's case, but don't bother asking the physician. As physicians, we are also at fault since we don't like talking about this either and may not invite your questions like we should. Your physician is there to give you their best advice, so please ask.

ICU Confidential In My Experience Edition: Time is the ultimate arbiter of what happens to you. Giving time to let the situation sink in. Giving time to ask the right questions and hear from the right sources. Giving time for natural emotional reactions to be balanced by rational thought. Giving time for your body to decide for us. I find that time, patience, and humility usually win the day, whatever winning means in your particular situation. This is not an excuse for being indecisive or supporting the status quo; it is a recognition that however much control you may want to have, time eventually decides for you.

F. Advanced Directives: Living Wills and Health Care Proxy

There are several legal documents called **advanced directives** that help define your wishes in regards to code status and other essential elements of your care. All patients are encouraged to complete these, optimally before they get too sick and definitely not in the heat of the moment. These documents outline your wishes should you become incapacitated and can't communicate them to your medical team in real time.

i. Living Will

This is the portion of advanced directives that lets your family and medical team know what you would or would not want to go through at the end of your life. It usually states that in the event of "a significant injury like severe brain damage, vegetative state, or other conditions where survival is not expected," you would or would not want life prolonging procedures, including **feeding tubes**, **CPR**, **mechanical ventilation**, and the like. It can also note a preference for treatments aimed at providing comfort even if these treatments would shorten your life. A living will has nothing to do with what you leave to whom!

ii. Medical Power of Attorney (POA)

Also part of advanced directives is a designation of a **health care proxy** or **surrogate**. This becomes your medical POA and is the person you name to make decisions on your behalf should you be unable to because you've become incapacitated. This person can be anyone you wish (providing they agree!). The medical POA does not have to be a family member.

If you do not name a health care proxy, most state laws deem your legal spouse as the default person making decisions on your behalf. If you have a "complicated" situation with your spouse, or they are someone you are separated from but still legally married to, the designation of health care proxy is even more consequential.

If you don't have a legal spouse, the law usually defers to your adult children in the absence of a designated health care proxy. With multiple children, the majority rules (hopefully you have an odd number of kids). I know you love all of them the same, but I also know you have a particular one in mind for this situation – name them and let everyone know ahead of time. It may be an awkward conversation, but it gets much worse later if you avoid it.

If you don't have children, you can likely retire earlier and do lots of traveling. As far as how this affects the default health care proxy, in the absence of children (or a legally recognized spouse), it's usually your parents' turn as decision makers.

Formally designating a health care surrogate (medical POA) becomes even more important if you feel the default designee does not know your current wishes or may not have your best interests in mind. This is especially true if your preferred health care proxy is not a family member or you have a complicated relationship with immediate family. An advanced directive will communicate this to your medical team should you be incapacitated.

iii. Organ Donor Designation

In some states, being designated as an organ donor also falls under advanced directives. Some states will indicate this on your driver's license, but most will look for a legal designation among these documents. We discuss organ procurement in greater detail below.

AARP® has a nice on-line resource linking living wills for each state: https://www.aarp.org/caregiving/financial-legal/free-printable-advance-directives/ or search AARP® Living Will forms by state.

ICU Confidential Final Destination Edition: Definitely take the time to review your advanced directives and discuss them with your family. If you already have a living will, discuss your wishes with your health care proxy and the rest of the family so they are aware of your wishes. You would be surprised at how devastating an already tragic situation can become when family members disagree about what they think you want or let their own wishes supersede yours. Solve this problem ahead of time by letting them know – it is *the most important gift you can give them.*

I would encourage everyone to learn what their family members would want for their end-of-life care as well. Talk to them and encourage them to complete their advanced directives. If they become suspicious that you are planning to kill them, just tell them you read it in this book, and it made all sorts of sense (you can even ask them to read this book if they need convincing).

ICU Confidential Final Destination 2 Edition: Although your health care proxy is not supposed to go against what you spell out in your living will, this quickly becomes a grey zone in practice. This is especially true when the living will is vague or unclear. I can't tell you how many times a spouse or a child has reversed a **DNR** order or requested a **feeding tube** be put in even when the living will noted otherwise. Whether it's guilt or difficulty coping, or the finality that is death, there is a difference between planning and executing.

While you may argue this is a legal document that must be followed, few physicians and even fewer hospital administrators will stand their ground when your health care proxy is belligerent and threatening a lawsuit and a call to local news. This is because most living wills leave room for interpretation (How can you be sure you won't recover? What if a miracle happens?). It's easier to give you a tracheostomy and a feeding tube, and transfer you to a long-term health facility where you (and your family) are someone else's problem.

Make sure your wishes are clear, and that you designate someone you trust to carry those wishes out even if they don't agree with them.

G. Organ Procurement

Deciding what will happen to your organs after you die is also a part of advanced directives. Organ donation (procurement) includes everything involved in donating (or someone obtaining) your organs when you die.

You may be surprised that the medical team that cares for you does not actually discuss this with you directly. The discussion is performed by a team of health care professionals that are independent of your care, and sometimes even your hospital. This separation is designed to eliminate any hint of bias on the part of the medical team caring for you – we're not just trying to kill you so we can harvest your organs (insert evil laugh here).

Organ donation is a standardized process that you may be involved in if you medically qualify as an organ donor (no active cancer, infection, etc.). Please note that this is very different from electively planning to donate a kidney to your uncle Joe.

> ***ICU Confidential Drivers's License Edition:*** Being designated as an organ donor on your driver's license does not affect how you are treated by paramedics or your hospital team. It is a very unfortunate urban myth that you may not get the same aggressive care or would be treated differently in some way. This makes no sense as the hospital cannot sell your organs. The designation only activates the asking of the organ donation question (which happens anyway) and is there to let your family know what your wishes may have been before you were hospitalized. This is carefully confirmed with you and your family if that time ever comes.

H. Defining Death

Most patients and physicians agree that death is defined by lack of life: no heartbeat + no breathing + no brain activity + eventually a funny smell = death. But there's some debate of what technically constitutes death if "all" of you is not dead.

Most everyone agrees that the complete lack of brain activity as determined by lack of blood flow to the brain, lack of electrical activity in the brain, lack of central reflexes, and so forth determines whether you are alive or not. This is defined as the **brain death** or **neurologic criteria** for death.

i. The Brain Death Definition

Brain death is medically defined as the complete and irreversible loss of all brain and brainstem function. This is determined by a set of strict criteria that when followed correctly guarantees confirmation that your brain function has permanently ceased. We make sure that medications, low oxygen, hypothermia, seizures, etc., are not fooling us, and the whole process is repeated and confirmed by a second independent expert (See Appendix II: Common Procedures in the ICU).

Once the brain dies, there is absolutely no hope for recovery even if the body can be kept alive through artificial means. The brain can never regenerate - the body will never have consciousness, will never breathe on its own, and the tissues will only survive through artificial means.

Brain death is by far the most widely accepted definition of death, ethically and legally. After all, no brain, no life. Right?

ii. Cardiopulmonary Death

There are circumstances where you've suffered an overwhelming stroke, had prolonged interruption of oxygen to the brain, or had severe head trauma, but your heart and lungs and other vital organs are still working. These neurologic conditions can lead to brain death, but your other organs are left intact, including the heart and the lungs. So, technically, the rest of your body is still "alive".

Because we can keep these organs functioning through the ventilator that breathes for you, with medications that keep the heart going, dialysis to replace the kidneys, and so on, there is a (very) small minority of people that define death by **cardio-pulmonary criteria** (also called **cardio-respiratory criteria**) alone. They believe that if the heart muscle functions, and any part of the body is still warm, you are still alive. This is based on the idea that if there's cell function anywhere in the body, you are not technically dead as a person. Some individuals invoke religious and other spiritual beliefs to support this.

iii. The Death Dilemma

Deviation from the brain death definition of death is typically the result of very tragic circumstances where the family cannot come to terms that their loved one's brain is no longer alive and that their body is basically a biological shell being kept functioning through artificial means. Think of kids with severe brain trauma or a young person who undergoes a prolonged cardiac arrest. It may be a lack of trust in the medical system and/or a profound misunderstanding of how biology works, feeling that we must have made a mistake as the body is still warm. This can evolve into months and sometimes years of full ventilator and other organ support at some facility in New Jersey (the first state to allow this), until the body succumbs to other medical complications.

Most states legally recognize brain death as death. At the time of this writing, only New Jersey allows death by cardio-pulmonary criteria to supersede brain death criteria. There have certainly been scenarios where your family categorically disagrees with the reality of brain death and makes a legal push to halt any disconnection from technologic support so that your body continues to function. In very rare cases, your body can even be moved to New Jersey (and possibly other states depending on when you read this) where a non-defined religious or spiritual objection to using the neurologic (brain death) criteria for death can be invoked. Your body will be kept alive artificially in an ICU or chronic ventilator facility until it succumbs to something else (like the Jersey Shore).

I think that a good way to approach this question is to ask: If we can keep a fully decapitated person's body "alive" with technology (not the head; that technology was only available in a weird movie from 1962), is the *person* alive? It's an awful and visceral example, but it drives home the point.

ICU Confidential Man Wakes Up from Coma After 20 Years Edition: Brain death is not at all the same as being in a coma. In a coma, your brain is very much alive, just unconscious (asleep without the ability to wake up). You can often breathe on your own, and have central reflexes, just not much else. Coma is *not* brain death and should not be confused for brain death.

ICU Confidential Take A Deep Breath Edition: If you have spontaneous respiration, you are not brain dead as the breathing reflex is initiated not in the spinal cord but in the brain. It doesn't mean you can breathe on your own, or that there is anything beyond only basic function, but it does mean the brain is alive.

ICU Confidential Posturing Edition: Significant brain damage may cause the body to exhibit a coordinated set of movements called **decorticate** and **decerebrate posturing**. The first looks like you're flexing both arms to your chest almost like you're fist bumping yourself. The second involves extending your wrists and elbows almost like you're imitating a penguin walking. Both involve extending your legs and ankles like a ballerina. These originate in the brain, so it means you're not brain dead. Both, however, suggest severe brain injury and a poor prognosis.

ICU Confidential Reflex Redux Edition: Remember when you went to the doctor as a kid, and they hit your knee with a small rubber hammer to make your leg jump? This is called a patellar reflex and is among a number of other **deep tendon reflexes** that are mediated by the spinal cord. The brain is not actually involved. Sometimes this can look like the person is moving. This obviously means the brain is not dead, right? Wrong. These types of reflexes don't need the brain as they are just part of an automatic electrical circuit between the muscles and the spinal cord. The critical care physician and the neurologist can tell these apart from movement triggered by brain activity.

11 What Happens After the ICU

So far, we've discussed many of the things that the ICU does, and all the interventions and specialists available there to make you better. This chapter is about how you leave the ICU, and what happens next.

A. Downgrades (A Good Thing!)

The term **downgrade** may sound like you are getting demoted. It's the opposite of an upgrade, after all – back to economy you go! But this is actually the best outcome in an ICU since you are getting better, enough to no longer need the ICU. I personally prefer the terms graduating or transitioning from the ICU.

Downgrades refer to a de-escalation of the type and complexity of help you require. As you get better, you need less monitoring, less specialized interventions, and fewer specialists to carry out these interventions. You are breathing on your own, maintaining safe blood pressure, and are awake enough to participate in your care. As you are downgrading (transitioning), you may be going to the regular hospital ward, the **telemetry** unit if heart monitoring is still required, or to an **intermediate care unit** that has a little more monitoring than telemetry but not nearly as much as the ICU. Leaving the ICU is a step closer to home. This is a good thing!

ICU Confidential You're Sending Me Back Edition: Transitioning out of the ICU can make patients nervous. You've just been closer to death than you would like, you're finally getting better, and now we want to send you out of the place where you got better. You may have felt that the conditions in the regular hospital ward are what made you worse in the first place, and now we're sending you back. We get that, and so my practice is to explain the goals that should be met for you to graduate from the ICU. We tick off the boxes as we meet those goals with the expectation that when we're ready, you're ready. You can certainly discuss your concerns with us; we will listen.

> ***ICU Confidential Miracle Edition:*** While rare, there are conditions where you can go home directly from the ICU. The typical scenario is when you are in the ICU for close monitoring after a high-risk procedure, like after **embolizing** a brain **aneurysm** or after a pacemaker insertion. We watch you for a set period of time during which complications are most likely and then have you go home. You may find it surprising that you would need to be in the ICU for extensive neurologic checks every hour for, say, 24 hours, but at 24 hours and 1 minute you can go straight home. This is a side effect of protocolized care, and works because it is based on extensive studies of patients with similar conditions.

B. Long Term Acute Care Hospitals (LTACH)

For prolonged stays for medical needs like **ventilator weening**, **wound care**, and severe **deconditioning** that require intense physical rehabilitation, you may still need the services of a hospital, but the resources (and mindset) of more chronic care. Therapies like IV medications, help with breathing, and other interventions that home or a nursing home is not able to provide may still be required, but the approach would be longer term and slower paced.

Long term acute care hospitals (LTACHs) assume that you will need up to another 30 days of care to continue your recovery. Some LTACHs provide an ICU level of care where respiratory therapists work with physicians to help slowly wean you from the ventilator. Some facilities can provide patients with additional needs like **dialysis** but may not have more advanced cardiac or neurologic support.

It's important to understand that the hospital is not giving up on you when you transfer to an LTACH. Rather, it's moving you to a place that more precisely meets your long-term needs. Think of the original ICU as the place we put the fire out, and the LTACH as the place where you rebuild. You wouldn't expect a firefighter to rebuild your burned-out kitchen any more than the kitchen contractor to put out your fire. LTACHs and rehabs are there to build you a new kitchen, with the many therapists and support staff to help make this happen.

ICU Confidential LTACH Edition: The quality of LTACHs varies greatly, even within the same corporate structure. Visiting the facility is highly recommended. Have your family meet with their representatives. They should pay special attention to how clean and nice the facility looks, what the staff looks like (clean uniforms, smiles on their faces, courtesy on display) and, most importantly, what the patients look like (do they look well cared for, kempt, comfortable). One of my patient's family members told me they make it a point to excuse themselves from the campus tour (say you need to use the restroom) and use the opportunity to take a quick look around on their own (while respecting the privacy of other patients). You should also ask for quality metrics – what is the rate of hospital acquired (**nosocomial**) infections, lower back (**sacral**) ulcers, falls, successful ventilator liberations, and the like.

ICU Confidential Not Giving Up Edition: I remember taking care of a young patient for very severe respiratory failure in the ICU. It was in the midst of the first wave of the COVID 19 pandemic. His lungs were badly damaged by inflammation and scarring and he spent many weeks on the ventilator fighting through a number of complications. When the worst of it was over, he was transferred to an LTACH where he could continue weaning from the ventilator and get his strength back through rehab. I saw him in my lung clinic about a year later. He was back at work, fully functional and looking well overall. It broke my heart when he recounted his story because he described the hospital as giving up on him when transitioning to an LTACH. Even though we fought tooth and nail to get him healthy enough for rehab, he saw it as giving up on him. That misunderstanding was clearly our fault because we failed to explain how and why it was time for the transition. If you are in this situation, know that transitioning to that next level of care is not the hospital giving up — it's that you've improved enough where you're ready to start rebuilding.

C. Nursing Homes and Chronic Ventilator Facilities

When there is little to no rehabilitation potential, and the expectation is that you have improved as much as you are going to and you still need extensive care, a nursing home or chronic ventilator facility is where you go. Depending on how well-resourced the facility is, the level of services can vary greatly. Knowing that you can't be taken care of at home, these places offer to keep you going with medical and rehabilitative services. Facilities with chronic ventilator beds are few and far between, and even if you are wealthy and/or have excellent long term care insurance, there never seem to be enough good facilities with available space.

> ***ICU Confidential Chronic Vent Edition:*** When you are beyond rebuilding, and have not made progress even in an LTACH, this becomes your life. You are kept alive by machines and/or you need too much help with basic activities of daily living like eating, going to the toilet, showering, or sometimes just breathing. These are often depressing situations, and places. Some are very nice, with staff who are very committed, and allow a better visitation environment, all while doing their best to provide some quality of life. Unfortunately, many become repositories for when you are stuck in medical purgatory. Available chronic ventilator facility beds are not common because reimbursement for this type of care is poor. Places that support patients with ventilators *and* dialysis are often even harder to find. In the absence of a chronic ventilator bed, you often end up spending many weeks or even months stuck in the ICU.

D. Home Care

I include home care as a destination because with enough resources and planning, it's actually pretty amazing what can be accomplished in your own home.

Once you are discharged from the ICU, there are many therapies that, with enough resources, can keep you at home. Ventilators, gastric tube pumps, and even IV therapies can be set up at home. Some patients can also have dialysis at home.

You must have the caregiver resources as well as the financial ones to make this happen. A lot of education has to go into home care, and a lot of commitment, as this can quickly become overwhelming for family and caregivers. Imagine what you would do in an emergency if the ventilator malfunctioned, or you have a mucus ball suddenly plugging up your airway, or if an IV line dislodges and now you're bleeding. Imagine if the feeding tube comes out. Even the most dedicated families need a lot of resources to manage this safely at home, and you have to be trained and prepared for these scenarios.

This does not apply to the *hospital at home* model where you are technically still "admitted" to the hospital with home equipment that measures and reports your vital signs, and medical personnel check in with you virtually. These programs are available in some medical institutions and may provide care for some patients that would otherwise have to be in the hospital ward. This usually applies for patients with relatively simple needs, like needing to complete a course of IV antibiotics. There is no ICU at home at present (except for that reclusive billionaire or crown prince).

E. End-of-Life Care

The social and medical care surrounding the actively dying process is referred to as end-of-life care. It includes things like pain and symptom control, help with toileting, nutrition, and the like. It includes important questions like where you want to be when you pass away, and how to get the staff and proper equipment to get you there. **Advanced directives** and **code status** are a major part of end-of life-care and were discussed in Chapter 10. Here we explore concepts life **palliative care, hospice,** and other services that are also part of the end-of-life care.

i. Palliative Care

The branch of medicine that focuses on relieving symptoms and stress in patients with severe illness is called palliative care. While palliative care is important in end-of-life care, it can also be provided at any stage of the medical journey.

Palliative care as a specialty includes **fellowship** training and **board certification** that qualifies skilled physicians who focus on ways to treat pain, anxiety, side effects of treatment, and other aspects of your serious illness. In the ICU, palliative care physicians assist with advanced directives and code status discussions and can take the time and perspective to discuss options like comfort measures only and hospice.

Palliative care can be offered in conjunction with disease-specific treatments. Hospice (see below) is the ultimate part of palliative care, when symptom relief becomes the only goal (also see Chapter 10: Code Status and More for additional information).

Palliative care physicians in the ICU serve as independent clinicians offering advice from a different perspective. In fact, studies show that patients who are also under the care of a palliative care physician not only have better symptom control but also live longer despite receiving *less* aggressive interventions at the end of life. Sometimes less really is more.

ii. Hospice

Contrary to many people's understandings, hospice is technically a medical plan and not a place. I would say the best description, however, is that hospice is a philosophy. The only requirement for enrollment is that you have a terminal medical condition with a life expectancy of less than 6 months. This can include obvious conditions like advanced cancer and heart failure, but also conditions like **dementia** and **failure to thrive**.

When the underlying disease is terminal and no longer treatable, or when the treatment is no longer acceptable to you as the patient, a transition to symptom focused care becomes a real alternative. Hospice is the framework that makes this alternative possible.

No more chemotherapy, blood draws, X-rays, or invasive procedures unless they are directly geared to providing comfort, like pain relief and relief from the many other symptoms of the disease. No more ventilators, pressors, advanced cardiac support, or all the IV lines and tubes. Hospice becomes a destination when the goal changes from *treat to cure* to *treat to comfort.*

Hospice can be initiated in the ICU room. If you are on a ventilator or requiring high doses of medications to support your blood pressure, and the expectation is that death will be imminent when these technologies are removed, we make sure you are comfortable before we start. Medications like narcotics (i.e. morphine) and benzodiazepines (i.e. midazolam) are provided to prevent air hunger, pain, and anxiety.

It is true that these medications can hasten death, but the intent is to make your passing as comfortable as possible. Your underlying terminal medical condition is what ends your life, not the medications. This is what distinguishes hospice from **euthanasia,** or physician assisted suicide. You pass comfortably from your underlying medical condition with your family or friends by your side.

If death is not imminent, most hospitals have private comfort centered rooms with throw pillows and calm music in the background. This is a less clinical environment with liberal visitation rights and lots of snacks. Your care is transferred to the hospice physician and nurse who meet your medical and spiritual needs (clergy and emotional support providers are also part of the package). If your passing is over weeks or longer, a hospice facility is an option. Hospice services at home can also be provided, but these are also resource intensive and require a significant amount of family support. Hospice at home is better suited to when the decline is expected to take weeks or longer.

> ***ICU Confidential Ask Me An Easier Question Edition:*** Enrolling into hospice is often a difficult decision. When your disease has reached a certain point, you no longer have control over what will ultimately happen – you will die from your disease. What you do have some control over is how you will spend the time you have left, and the form that death will take – in the hospital hooked up to machines and undergoing invasive procedures to the end, or at home surrounded by family as you slip into a deep sleep. The key is recognizing when that time has come, hopefully not too early, and not too late.

iii. Compassionate Removal of Technological Support or De-escalation of Care

If you are already on a ventilator, pressors, advanced cardiac support, and/or other life support interventions, and you decide to transition to comfort measures only or to hospice, there is a process to remove this support. Such de-escalation is done in a way that minimizes any pain or discomfort, including anticipating and pretreating you to more gently transition from, for example, being on a ventilator to breathing on your own.

De-escalation of care medically speaking means you've gotten to the point where your goals of care are to focus on comfort rather than trying to fix an unfixable disease, and to remove any forms of life support without causing pain or discomfort. Removing a patient from life support is not considered a procedure, but there are many things involved in doing this correctly, and we understandably get a lot of questions about this.

If you are on a ventilator and are already showing signs of considerable discomfort when we try and wake you up, we usually continue a low dose sedative as we take you through the process. The respiratory therapist will perform a deep suction, deflate the endotracheal tube cuff, and remove the breathing tube. They may place an oxygen cannula or mask for comfort, even if it's only providing a small amount of oxygen or humidified air. If you are showing any signs of distress, more medication is provided until you appear comfortable.

For pressors and cardiac assist devices, these are typically titrated down to their lowest level of support, then turned off and removed if that is your wish. We try and leave you in as natural a state as possible while keeping you comfortable and letting your body do whatever it will naturally do. The medications used to keep you comfortable include narcotics to relieve pain and benzodiazepines to prevent anxiety. These are titrated according to your symptoms.

ICU Confidential How Long Will It Be Edition: How quickly you pass away depends on many different factors. I typically tell my patients (or their family members) that it may be minutes to days. If you're dying from a stroke but your lungs and heart are okay, you may be in a coma for some days to come. If you are dying from heart failure or severe shock, de-escalating your pressors may be a rapid terminal event. No matter how long it may be, our goal in this scenario is to make sure you are as comfortable and as natural as possible through the dying process.

iv. Physician Assisted Suicide / Euthanasia:

In the United States, select states have a legally sanctioned process for you to end your own life under medical supervision. You must be in the final stages of a terminal illness causing unbearable and untreatable distress and have made a conscious decision that staying alive is no longer acceptable.

Each state has its own set of rules, but the process generally involves confirmation by a number of professionals. Aside from your physician, you will also likely be speaking with the ethics committee member, and a mental health specialist to make sure you have the capacity to make this decision (i.e. have your full faculties about you.

While there are many safeguards in place, this remains a complicated and controversial issue. If you are in a state where this is legal and wish to know more about what is involved, please speak to your intensivist and case manager.

> ***ICU Confidential What's the Difference Edition*:** Physician assisted suicide is not considered the same as compassionate removal of technology, or not providing this technology in the first place (i.e. **DNR**). In these scenarios, you pass away directly from your disease. That is, if not for your disease, removing life support would not result in your immediate death. In physician assisted suicide, while you may eventually die from your disease, what ends your life in the moment are medications specifically administered to stop your breathing and your heart.

> ***ICU Confidential Can't I Have It All Edition:*** Why can't physicians control all the discomfort *and* treat the underlying illness at the same time? When you are fighting the illness, this is certainly the intent. The question is: what if the two goals contradict each other? When the underlying illness gives unrelenting pain, but you can't give enough pain medication because it may stop your breathing, the pain control has to give way. When chemotherapy makes you so sick you want to die despite nausea and vomiting medications, then that's the price of therapy because the goal is to fight the cancer. Unfortunately, while we do everything possible to make you comfortable, the effects of the underlying illness and the side effects of the therapy can't always be controlled.

> ***ICU Confidential He's a Fighter Edition:*** Many people see their medical journey as a battle against their disease. They wage war on their cancer, they battle their heart failure, they attack their emphysema. When an illness becomes clearly terminal, it is important to recognize that you don't stop fighting, *you change what you are fighting for.* Your battle now becomes getting your symptoms under control, being able to go home if that is your wish, and passing away on your own terms.

F. ICU Purgatory

When you are too sick to leave the ICU but are not immediately dying, and your goals are to continue treatment, you effectively live at the ICU Hotel (*0* stars on Tripadvisor®). There are different scenarios in which you can get stuck in the ICU for long periods of time. One involves an inability to wean from the ventilator. You may also have a slowly progressive terminal illness like cancer or heart failure or COPD where you recover from an acute exacerbation but not to the point of being able to leave the ICU.

There may be no beds that can meet your needs at a long-term acute care hospital, or you may have other issues that prevent you from transfer, like being on continuous (around the clock) hemodialysis, or not having rehabilitation potential, or no insurance. This can also happen with end stage liver or heart failure, where you can't live without advanced therapies usually in the form of continuous IV drips or intravascular devices that keep you going but need continuous ICU monitoring. You can't leave the ICU because of the type of support you are getting, and organ failure is progressing at a pace of weeks, not hours.

Being stuck in the ICU can also happen if you are an organ transplant candidate, but no transplant is available, so you wait and wait. If you need a transplant but do not qualify because you're still drinking alcohol or are too old or have too many other organs impaired, you end up too sick to leave the ICU with no way forward.

Another reason patients get stuck in the ICU is when they need a chronic ventilator facility, but there are no available beds, or you have no insurance to pay. There is an on-going shortage of beds in facilities that can handle chronic but complex medical needs such as ventilator support along with dialysis along with heart sustaining IV infusions. The ICU becomes your home until you get better (sometimes), or you decompensate further and die (most times).

G. End-Stage Cancer and the ICU

Cancer carries many complications that become more severe and common as the disease advances. The local effects of the cancer pushing on or eating through vital structures like blood vessels, bones, and organs presents one set of issues, but the overall effects on your immune system, blood coagulation, and frailty are what usually kill you. Overwhelming infection (sepsis), blood clots going to the lungs or brain, heart attacks, and metastatic disease where the cancer physically spreads to different organs causing them to shut down top the list.

Cancer treatments often carry significant side effects as well. Chemotherapy wipes out your immune system leaving you susceptible to infection. Immunotherapy can cause an auto-immune (allergic) reaction that attacks your body, especially the lungs. Radiation therapy can cause burns and scarring in your organs. All this is more than worth it if it cures your cancer and/or gives you substantially more time and quality of life, and the ICU is the place to deal with these complications when they get that bad.

Fortunately, amazing advances in cancer treatments have improved cure rates and have provided more (quality) time for patients. These advances have rightfully created significant hope for patients and families. Unfortunately, they sometimes create unrealistic expectations as well. There remain many cancers that, despite all our knowledge and technology, remain incurable and consume the patient in the worst ways.

A profoundly tragic scenario that we see in the ICU is cancer that is already very far advanced, usually despite multiple rounds of chemo and immunotherapy, radiation, and surgery. Sometimes this is a brand new diagnosis but already too far gone to treat. All too often, the ICU becomes a repository for patients dying of cancer that is well past this point of no return. These patients are often beyond any additional treatment options but are not ready to let go (or more typically, their family isn't).

Sooner or later, a medical complication makes them acutely sick to the point of needing ICU care. We take care of the sepsis or blood clot or stroke or whatever other complication made you acutely decompensate, but we cannot fix the underlying problem — the cancer itself. The catch-22 is that even if there was another treatment option, you need to be healthy enough to survive it, which is not possible due to the cancer complications themselves.

An advanced cancer patient, especially if they are young, can remain on the ventilator or the myriads of other support technologies in the ICU for weeks. All this continues while the cancer slowly eats away at you. Eventually, you have a complication that you do not recover from, despite all our efforts.

> ***ICU Confidential Why Me Edition:*** The tragic scenario that is dying of cancer in the ICU is often a result of the terrible stress you and your loved ones are going through, and the natural desire not to talk about death as if not talking about it can somehow prevent it. This is often seen in younger patients where it is incomprehensible that nothing more can be done to treat the cancer. This creates a terrible, unfair situation. There is no justice in cancer; looking for it will drive you crazy and rob you of what peace and time you have remaining.

H. Death

The unbreakable law of death is often expressed in the setting of the ICU. Whether after multiple attempts at resuscitation, or death through natural means, once you pass away, a number of protocols are in place to manage what happens next.

First, when you pass away, the clinician is required to do a declaration of death. This involves a brief exam consisting of listening for a heartbeat and checking for pulses, breathing and basic reflexes. The physician also documents time of death. The body is then released to the coroner.

We typically give the family time to say goodbye at the bedside before the body is transferred to the morgue where the cold will slow decomposition. The funeral home of your choice is then contacted; they pick up the body as you make funeral arrangements. If there is any possibility of foul play, the body is not released to the funeral home until the **medical examiner** does their examination, including a through autopsy if required (see below).

Declaration of brain death when the heart and/or lungs are still functioning with or without support presents a different scenario (see Appendix II Common Procedures In the ICU). To date, there have not been any cases when the brain death protocol was strictly adhered to and then the patient "came back to life."

Keep in mind, brain death does not apply to being in a coma or a persistent vegetative state where the brain function is highly limited and/or the patient is unconscious, but the brain is still alive. Those are very different scenarios from brain death.

I. Death Certificate:

The death certificate is a legal document submitted to the **medical examiner** (ME) and the **Bureau of Vital Statistics** and is legally required after you or your loved one passes away. Among other things, it notes time of death, records if death was natural or not, and explains the cause of death (the why). The *why* is listed in a causative way (A as a result of B as a result of C) with an approximate duration (hours, weeks, etc.).

Other contributing medical issues are also listed. The death certificate is signed by your intensivist when you die in the ICU, the hospitalist if on the ward, and usually your primary care provider if at home. If it becomes a medical examiner case, such as if foul play is suspected, the ME signs it after examining your body.

The death certificate usually takes a day or two to be generated and has to make it back to the physician before they can complete and submit it. This sometimes means it ends up in the hands of a physician on duty at that time, possibly someone you've never met. They fill it out based on information in your hospital notes. The death certificate is faxed or emailed to the funeral home and the Bureau of Vital Statistics. The funeral home needs it to be completed before burial or cremation.

> ***ICU Confidential Contributing Conditions Edition:*** There are often legal consequences of what is on the death certificate in the form of disability or other payments due the surviving spouse. For example, if someone dies of a heart attack and they have diabetes, a known risk factor for heart disease, it's important that this be listed under contributing medical issues. Why? If you happen to have a military service connection (for example, Agent Orange exposure through the Veteran's Administration) or are part of a class action lawsuit (like asbestos or talc), this may affect if your beneficiaries get paid. Make sure they discuss this with the physician doing the death certificate so they can be as complete as possible.

> ***ICU Confidential SVU Edition:*** The death certificate is often an estimate or best guess of what happened to you. This is especially true when you die at home and your primary care physician must estimate cause of death based on your medical history. Unless the police suspect foul play, the cause of death is just your physician's best guess based on your medical history and the case may not get referred to the medical examiner.

J. Autopsy:

An autopsy is a medical procedure where a physician specially trained in determining the cause of death (**pathologist**) performs a comprehensive examination of the corpse, both externally and internally. They carefully examine the body for bruises and other signs of foul play. They then cut the body open in a protocolized way, dissect out the organs, and help determine and/or confirm a cause of death. This is legally triggered if you've died under unclear circumstances where foul play is suspected (the pathologist in that scenario is the medical examiner or forensic pathologist).

If a patient's death is unexplained, an autopsy can also assist in finding the answer. If your family suspects that your death was a result of malpractice, they may request an autopsy as well. This can be done at the hospital or by an independent pathologist. The hospital is bound to honor this request, but not to pay for it – that will be your family's responsibility.

12 Advice for Getting the Best Experience:

Eating, Sleeping, Exercising, Going to the Bathroom, and Staying Sane in the ICU

Understanding your ICU environment, including why you're there, who's who, what's happening around you, what the procedures are, and so on, are key elements to getting what you need in the best manner possible (if only you had some insider information). When it comes down to it, it's what you do with this information, and how you interact with the ICU staff, that really makes the difference.

Once you are no longer at the precipice of death, you often transition into a more prolonged therapy stage. It's imperative that once you are acutely stabilized (awake, breathing on your own, able to eat) you don't forget, or let us forget, the essential day-to-day activities that you need to continue your recovery. I'm talking about basics – eating, using the bathroom, exercising, sleeping, and the like. These are the things that will make you feel a little closer to normal again.

This can take anywhere from a few days to a week or longer. As ICU physicians, we tend to have a SWAT team mentality where we make big things happen in an emergency. But we also realize that to keep things going, we can't forget about all these regular day-to-day things that keep you on the road to recovery and prevent you from becoming an emergency again.

A. Eating and Nutrition

In the throes of a ground invasion, a turkey sandwich is not top of mind. But once you've been in the foxhole for a while, it starts sounding pretty good. Medically speaking, your body can be okay without food for up to 5 to 7 days, as long as we keep you hydrated and keep your electrolytes in check. We do try to feed you as soon as possible, and we know the gut is the best way to do this.

If you are too sick to eat on your own, we give you formula through a **nasogastric** or **orogastric tube** going through your nose or mouth respectively into the stomach (see Appendix I: Machines and Things).

If we can't get your gut to work, like after bowel surgery, or due to certain medications (like high doses of **pressors**), or if your gut just refuses to work (**ileus**), we start talking about feeding you directly through your bloodstream. This is called **Partial Parenteral Nutrition** (**PPN**) or **Total Parenteral Nutrition** (**TPN**). PPN only requires a peripheral **IV** and while useful cannot meet all your nutritional needs. TPN requires a **central line** and is designed to fully replace your nutritional needs (see Appendix II: Procedures Common in the ICU).

Nutrition through your veins increases the risk of a number of complications. These include pancreatitis and gallbladder problems, infections including fungus in your blood (**fungemia**, bad news), and needing a separate central line. This is in part why we tend to wait as long as possible to go to this option. Despite all the advances in the chemistry of nutrition, nothing is as good as using your own gut. Even when your gut is doing fine, you are often prevented from eating because you are waiting for a specific test or procedure.

Anything that requires sedation will require you to fast before the procedure to make anesthesia safer (so you don't throw up and aspirate your stomach contents into your lungs). This often leads to many hours of skipped meals or tube feeds being on hold.

The ICU is notorious for not keeping up with your nutrition. Make sure your medical team is reminded that you're hungry and that your nutrition is important, even if that means eating dinner at 10 pm or increasing the tube feed rate to compensate for the pauses. Don't be shy about letting us know if we are keeping you from food too long. We also encourage your family to bring food that may be more appealing to you; please do ask us first since your medical condition may require certain dietary restriction.

> ***ICU Confidential Don't (Force) Feed Me Edition:*** When you are acutely sick, your appetite tends to shut down. This is also true when you are chronically ill with what we refer to as **failure to thrive**. You just stop being hungry and stop eating; your body may be slowly shutting down and stops asking for food. Force-feeding you in these situations is very uncomfortable and is not going to save your life. Artificial feeding is considered a form of life support, and you can elect to withhold it.

B. Going to the Bathroom

As we learn in kindergarten, everybody poops. But when the body is in shock and fighting for its life, the gut goes quiet. The medications we give to keep you comfortable on a ventilator or to control your pain, and the lack of mobility, can also lead to severe constipation. On the other hand, sometimes you have the opposite problem, especially if you're being fed formula through a gastric tube.

In any event, we need to make sure you stay regulated. As such, moving your bowels is part of the **ICU bundle** where we check your bowel and urine status every day and usually have you on what we call a **bowel regimen**. This consists of things like fiber supplements, stool softeners, and more. If you have a certain routine that includes these supplements, let us know so we can start them before a problem develops. Even if you're not eating much, you are constantly producing mucus and secretions and sloughing cells in your gastrointestinal tract that will form stool.

If you have diarrhea, we check for gut infections, adjust the tube feed formulas, and give you medications to slow down your gut. We also work to protect your skin and make sure we keep pressure off sensitive areas.

Urinating is equally important. If you have urinary retention due to an enlarged prostate or a bladder problem, or we need to precisely monitor how much you urinate, you may need a urinary catheter. We work to get it out as soon as possible to help avoid infection and discomfort. If you are having trouble with incontinence, we have external devices that are safe and hygienic (condom or wick applications).

Please don't be afraid to voice your concerns – this is the most important thing you can do. We can add or remove certain medications, mobilize your body with help from your nurse and physical therapy, and address problems early so they don't turn into serious complications. Please don't be embarrassed – we are here to help in *every* way.

> ***ICU Confidential Let It Go Edition:*** Severe constipation can be very uncomfortable, and also lead to vomiting, malnutrition, and even a surgical emergency. We keep you on a bowel regimen, sometimes including suppositories and enemas. In bad situations, we manually disimpact you. The disimpaction is usually done by the most junior member of the medical team.

> ***ICU Confidential Keep It In Edition:*** Significant diarrhea can also ruin your otherwise lovely ICU experience. This can happen from antibiotics and other medications, from a terrible gut infection called **C. diff** (**Clostridioides difficile**), from bleeding in your GI track, and from bowel surgery. Sometimes it's because your anti-constipation medications weren't discontinued in a timely manner after you finally did go (that's on us!). Diarrhea in the ICU can be uncomfortable and dangerous, leading to skin breakdown and possible infection in very sensitive areas, as well as dehydration and electrolyte disturbances. Sometimes when diarrhea is extensive and can't be controlled, a rectal tube made from silicone and plastic is used by placing it in, well, you know.

C. Sleeping

Sleep is essential to your mental, neurological, immune, cardiac, and other basic functions. And, good sleep actually makes you *feel* good! In the ICU, good quality sleep is both important and exceedingly hard to come by.

As your condition improves, you may no longer need heavy-duty pain and sedative medications. Once you are conscious again, you may still be stuck in bed and bored out of your mind. Your sleep-wake cycle is already disrupted, and you may start having insomnia. To make it even worse, we seem to wait until you finally fall asleep to check your vitals, draw blood, and otherwise interrupt your rest. It's usually noisy too, between the IV pumps beeping, machine alarms going off, and the drama unfolding in the hall and neighboring rooms.

We encourage you to be active during the day, getting the window shades up, getting your sudoku on, and staying awake as much as possible to build up your sleep drive for the nighttime. While difficult to enforce, we do employ evening quite hours to minimize disturbing your sleep. Sleeping aids are frowned upon although we sometimes use melatonin to keep your body clock ticking.

There are some well-known complications of being in the ICU, and not being able to sleep is a big one. It will literally drive you crazy (**delirious**).

ICU Confidential Confused About Confusion Edition: If you do find yourself getting more confused, it may be the poor sleep or it may be a side effect of medication or your medical condition. While we evaluate you on an on-going basis, including checking on your mental status, we may not be aware of your cognitive baseline (and sometimes people can hide deficits pretty well). Please let us know so we can work on figuring it out – don't be embarrassed to tell us you're feeling confused.

D. Exercising

Now that your immediate life-threatening emergency has been resolved, it's time to build your strength back up. We're not talking about pull-ups and burpees. Exercise in the ICU setting means sitting at the edge of the bed, being able to bear weight, and transitioning to the recliner. These are actually big deals, and you should be proud of yourself for being able to do this. When you're ready, you will gradually start to walk, including doing laps around the ICU hallway.

Getting physically active as soon as possible during your recovery has been found to prevent delirium, bed sores, pain, constipation, and deconditioning. It also just makes you feel more human. Please don't try this alone – you are hooked up to way too many wires, tubes and IVs. Make sure the nurse and/or the physical therapist are there to ensure a safe "work-out."

ICU Confidential a Little Goes a Long Way Edition: Getting physical is a quality marker in the ICU. Even if you can't do much, turning you every 2 hours is an important way to prevent bed sores and muscle pain. It's not easy if you're in pain or trying to rest, and you may not be too happy about it at the moment, but hopefully you'll thank us later.

E. Maintaining Mental Health

Mix in being very sick, a slew of medications and procedures, and lack of sleep, and it's no wonder it's so easy to become disoriented in the ICU. Your consciousness and level of alertness can wax and wane. We call this **delirium**. It can be pretty scary to feel this way or to see your loved one so confused, but it is temporary; it's not the same as **dementia**.

Your brain will come back to normal as things settle down.

We try and help by minimizing the sedatives and hypnotics or using short-acting versions and then only when absolutely necessary. We try to keep your sleep-wake cycle intact. We try to keep up with your nutrition and generally get you healthy enough to graduate from the ICU. Remember, as hard as it is feeling confused, or seeing your loved one in this state, delirium will improve with recovery and time.

Delirium can also indicate a new medical problem. This can be the first sign of infection, especially in older people, as well as a sign of other neurological events. Your physician should look at all the possibilities.

Being sick can make you consistently confused as well. Our neurologists call this **toxic encephalopathy**. This is a diagnosis given to explain your confusion once all the other reasons are ruled out, like stroke, brain infection, brain tumor, and so forth. This should also improve as your overall health recovers.

It is also not uncommon to experience significant anxiety and depression in the ICU. You can help maintain your mental health through this medical crisis by staying optimistic and focusing on every success, no matter how small. You participated in physical therapy today, excellent! You ate a little bit more today than yesterday, fantastic! You had a bowel movement, let's celebrate!

You can also optimize your mental health by engaging with your family and friends. You can connect through video calling, watch something interesting on-line, catch up on your reading (hint, hint), and otherwise distract yourself in healthy ways. Your body may be stuck in bed all day, but you can help your mind escape your room through communication and technology (just make sure it comes back).

Perhaps most importantly, if feelings of anxiety or depression start to overwhelm you, please don't try and ignore them - just let us know. Most ICUs have social workers and even psychologists who can talk you through your feelings and suggest ways to cope. Sometimes, just having someone listen to what you're going through can make all the difference.

> ***ICU Confidential Dazed and Confused Edition:*** Delirium by definition is reversible. However, patients that get delirious are at higher risk for other complications. These include falls, becoming combative, and requiring restraints. This, of course, makes you even more delirious. Having delirium in the hospital also increases the risk of being diagnosed with dementia down the road (long after you leave the hospital).

F. Keeping Up With Life Outside the ICU

The rest of life doesn't stop just because yours almost did. When you first get sick, it may be without warning giving you no time to prepare. You may need to figure out how to handle work and family in a hurry. As hours become days, all the normal things that have to be taken care of start to pile up as well. There's the yard, the mail, the pets. There are also the bills, the calls you have to make, and don't forget about work.

Hopefully, you have a social network capable of taking this off your plate. It's always a good idea to think of this ahead of time. Maybe consider what you would do if you were to travel for a week or two. Who would take care of these things? If you live alone, planning is even more essential. Even in a shared household tasks are often delineated by individuals (I don't pay the bills; my spouse doesn't climb a ladder). For all of us, having a plan for emergencies is a good idea. You don't have to cross-train in every task – just make sure your backup knows where you keep the extra house key, and where the ladder is.

G. Dealing With Insurance

Having to eventually pay the hospital bill typically means dealing with insurance. Fortunately, the hospital is kind enough to check on this for you right away, starting from when you called 911, I think (a joke, the 911 operator does not notify your insurance, as far as we know). Shortly after you check into the ER, you will be visited by a helpful individual with a computer tablet or computer on wheels. They will take your demographic information and your insurance information.

You will subsequently be visited by a social worker and/or case manager. They can clarify your benefits and are there to make sure your insurance is there for them, I mean for you. Although they are there to advocate for the hospital, your goals typically align, and they will fight to make sure they get you all your benefits. You may even get a call from your insurance directly in which case be honest about what you know but also what you may not know and direct them to the case manager.

Some insurance companies also require you to file a claim as you are getting ready for discharge. Make sure to discuss whatever steps you may need to take with your case manager.

In the ICU, insurance does not typically play a role in the acute process of saving your life. As ICU physicians, we don't know what insurance you have, or even if you have insurance. We do what has to be done to treat your critical illness and don't let the insurance question guide our medical decisions; we let the hospital administration deal with the financial part.

Insurance may make a difference, however, if you need an organ transplant or a very expensive medication or procedure that can be classified as elective. It definitely makes a difference if you need a special rehabilitation or other facility after the ICU.

> ***ICU Confidential How Much is That Appendix in the Window Edition:*** There are countless scenarios where pricing will vary considerably depending on your insurance or lack thereof, where you're getting your care, who is taking care of you, and how things are documented. In practice, pricing is typically pre-negotiated well ahead of time and is likely competitive; otherwise, your insurance would not be accepted at that hospital. Your physician will have no idea and will refer you to the case manager. You are always within your rights to ask questions about the cost of your care and get these questions answered.

> ***ICU Confidential Getting Insurance While Hospitalized Edition:*** If you are not insured when you land in the hospital, you may think getting insurance is as impossible as getting hurricane insurance when you're already in the middle of a storm. Except, not: if you qualify for government insurance programs like Medicaid or Medicare, the case manager may be able to get you enrolled while you are actually in the hospital. This process often takes time and lots of paperwork, but it may be required if you don't want to be stuck in medical purgatory

or with insurmountable medical debt. This often occurs when you are beyond the acute illness but are not healthy enough for home and are looking for a rehab or long-term acute care hospital.

Sometimes, you need to go in the opposite direction and escalate your care, as in the case of needing a special treatment, surgery, or organ transplant. No insurance, no transfer, no transplant. Sometimes, it's just getting your medications covered after discharge. Use your case manager to help you clarify your options. In my experience, once you are discharged it is effectively much harder to get this kind of help.

H. Interacting With Your Medical Team: Be the Person Your Mom Thinks You Are

Just as there are expectations of how we as physicians should be communicating with the patient and their family – professionalism, respect, patience, and kindness – we have expectations of how communication should happen from the patient and family end. Interestingly, when we run into friction, it is more often with family and friends rather than the patient themselves (kind of like coaching kids sports – the kids are great, the parents, not so much).

What follows are some commonsense pieces of advice, for patients and family members, as to how to interact with your ICU team members and get the best results.

i. Be Nice:

In the ICU, as elsewhere, it helps to be kind, appreciative, and patient. In other words, treat others like you would like to be treated. Don't get me wrong; this doesn't mean you don't advocate for yourself - make sure your concerns are heard. It just means please do so in a respectful way. Assume the best and give people the benefit of the doubt. They don't necessarily know your journey, and that you've told your story 8 times to 8 different people in the past 2 hours, and that you're in pain, and that you may be panicked and overwhelmed. Being nice will pay dividends. This is also the same advice I give to the physicians I train – treat patients with respect, humility, and niceness, and give each patient the benefit of the doubt, even if it's the 8th patient they've seen in the past 2 hours.

ii. Be There:

This is for family and friends: being present at the bedside for your loved one goes a long way to good communication, in both directions. Not only can you inform us of some special element of the patient's history, but we can inform you directly of what is going on and why. This prevents a lot of miscommunications.

It also allows you to directly see how your loved one is doing, including seeing details like their X-rays and CT scans — I show these to every family during rounds — and get your questions answered in real time. It also shows us that you care. This is important because your medical team is influenced by the same push and pull of human nature as everyone else, and if we see that you are involved and caring, we can't help but take a little extra time and join you in that effort.

Please remember, however, that it is most helpful to have (only) one or two people as the family representatives who can help disseminate information to the rest of your loved ones, and bring their questions to us directly, limiting repetition and unnecessary anxiety.

iii. Talk to Us Like You Know Something We Don't:

While we approach your care from a vantage point of what works for most people, you may not be most people. If you had an unexpected reaction to a particular medication, speak up and let us know. If you had a particular experience that informs your choices for a procedure or intervention, talk to us and help us understand. Just do so in a nice way and I promise we will accommodate.

iv. Talk to Us Like We Know Something You Don't:

It is perfectly reasonable to expect your questions to be answered but please start with assuming your medical team is coming from a place of knowledge and experience that is more informed than yours (unless you are also a physician with relevant expertise). Google® and AI may sound convincing, but they are far from perfect (for now). There is also a fine line between asking for an explanation and dictating your own care.

This also applies to the expectation that we should take you through medical school. We do try to explain how the body works so that you have a clear understanding of the mechanisms of your disease, but there is a limit. Most of us will have the capacity for patience, and we will take the time to stop and explain, but we do need time to actually take care of you and all our other patients.

Having said this, my expectation is that you will not blindly follow medical (or any other) advice, and the better informed you are, the easier our conversation becomes. To learn more about your medical conditions, it's imperative to go to well validated sources that reflect medical science, not medical bias; see the next section for some suggestions.

I. Educating Yourself On Your Condition

We want you to trust us. The best way for that to happen is to make sure you're well informed. It's kind of like going to a mechanic and being told you need a new alternator. If you knew what that was and what kind of problems it gives you, you could better trust the mechanic's recommendations. Otherwise, you just have to take their word for it and maybe leave the shop with an uneasy feeling. Your health is more important than your car. When researching your medical issues, please get informed by going to reputable sources, and always consider who funds these sources and how they are vetted. Here's a few tips you might find helpful:

i. National Medical Society's Guidelines and Recommendations Websites: YES!

Many of these organizations have excellent patient-centered websites and other resources designed to provide information directly to patients and not just physicians. These are the primary sources for most reputable health systems and other medical websites. They can be hard to navigate but are worth it.

Make sure you're on a real organization's site and not one that sounds important but is only trying to sell you something. Also, keep in mind that for information to be included in guidelines it has to be fully vetted and time tested. This means the information is more reliable but may also not include the most recent *hot-off-the-press* developments.

Some prestigious medical journals have also created patient-centered resources. They are generally very well vetted and trusted by healthcare professionals, and may also include information on more recent developments.

Some examples of medical organizations are: The American Medical Association, American College of Physicians, Society of Critical Care Medicine, American College of Chest Physicians, American Thoracic Society, the American Academy of Pediatrics.

Some examples of major medical journals with excellent patient centered resources include: New England Journal of Medicine (NEJM), Journal of the American Medical Association (JAMA), and the Lancet.

ii. A General Site from a Reputable Medical Center: YES!

These sites have general information that helps you learn about a particular disease, test, or treatment. They usually don't go into a great amount of detail, but they are reviewed and checked for accuracy.

Some examples include: Mayo Clinic, Cleveland Clinic, Johns Hopkins Medicine, Mass General Brigham, Stanford Health Care, and many more.

iii. Any Site That Tries to Sell You Something: NO!

Whether it's the latest cure or the must try gadget, anything that asks you to buy something is a hard no. This usually includes remedies that sound too good to be true, because they are, even if they are being sold on a slick website fronted by someone in a white coat. These are scammers trying to take advantage of your anxiety and desperation.

iv. Sites That Have Been Around For a While and Have a Reasonable Reputation – YES! (*qualified*)

These sites have general information about your symptoms or conditions. They do provide advertising and sometimes links trying to sell you something, so buyers beware. Be careful not to fall down the rabbit hole when doing this type of research into your symptoms. Ask an actual health professional. (Also, if you have rabbit holes big enough for you to fall into, those weren't made by rabbits.)

Some examples include: WebMD®, Healthline®, and Merck Manual.

v. Anything on X® (fka Twitter), Tik Tok®, YouTube® and the Like: NO! NO! Triple NO!

None of these platforms require an individual to have any credentials to post about healthcare (or anything else). If a channel is run by any of the "YES" organizations, they may be credible, but you have to confirm the source.

There are also physicians and other professionals on these platforms who may be trying to be a balance to all the misinformation, but they must be vetted too (anyone can buy scrubs and a white coat).

In the overwhelming majority of cases, however, you might as well be taking advice from your cousin's friend's neighbor's hairdresser, someone who at best does not have any clue as to what medical advice they are about to offer and at worst is deliberately spreading disinformation to attract followers. Poo, poo, poo.

vi. Artificial Intelligence/ChatABC – NO! (or, *Not Yet*)

The current level of artificial intelligence depends on algorithms that scour vast amounts of data from the internet and proprietary databases and compile this data to offer seemingly professional sounding advice. The main issue, of course, is the validity of that data to begin with. The phrase garbage in, garbage (dangerous advice) out comes to mind. Given the rate of learning, however, this is expected to improve tremendously, but until then, reader beware.

vii. Disease Specific Organizations - YES!

Many of these organizations are founded by patients and families. Not only can they give good advice, but they often have support groups and resources to participate in research. Always do your due diligence and consider who funds these organizations and if they are trying to sell you something.

Examples include: The American Lung Association, Pulmonary Fibrosis Foundation, Surviving Sepsis Campaign, Extracorporeal Life Support Organization (ELSO).

viii. The Government: YES/NO/MAYBE?:

The government runs a number of reputable, if sometimes difficult to navigate, medical websites, especially at the federal level. Examples include MedlinePlus (from the National Library of Medicine), Centers for Disease Control and Prevention (CDC), National Institutes of Health (NIH), and the Food and Drug Administration (FDA). They provide medical facts accepted by the general medical community. They are made up of real people with real knowledge. However, as I write this in late 2025, a major disclaimer (below) needs to be included.

Until very recently, the government-run websites mentioned above would have been the gold standard of medical information. Unfortunately, while non-medical beliefs have always had some influence in medicine, this has now really affected the quality of information patients may receive. If your local or state or federal health department is at odds with the medical societies that specialize in that medical problem, this should be a warning sign that the government agency advice should be handled with care.

You should absolutely engage with your physician to help explain any discrepancies you find. It's perfectly fine to challenge your physician with this information; we will do our best to explain any differences in opinion.

> ***ICU Confidential Doctors Can Be Criminals Too Edition:*** If you try hard enough, you can usually find someone with a medical degree to sell you what you're looking for. The more desperate the situation and the more you're willing to pay, the more likely you'll find someone who is trying to take advantage of you. At best these so-called professionals are ignorant or contrarian, at worst they are just plain criminals. If 99.99% of physicians interpret the available medical information in the same way, they are in that moment correct. The chance that the one individual who buys a website and sells you a miracle cure is right, and everyone else is wrong is exactly 0.0000%. When it comes to your health, don't replace research and science with fear and desperation, and don't fund the next Ferrari® of an online scammer.

ix. Sources Where Physicians Go For Information: MAYBE!

I remember in my fancy medical school one of our first lectures was by C. Everett Coop, a former US Surgeon General. In it, he highlighted the sheer volume of medical information and how it was expanding exponentially. He emphasized that knowing how to find and scrutinize information was as important as knowing it in the first place. This was prophetic, before smart phones even existed!

As physicians, our go-to sources for rapid and dependable information include **PubMed**®, **UpToDate**®, **Epocrates**®, and others. For clinical trials, we access **Clinicaltrials.gov**, a searchable database for all active research trials in the US. This information is generally well vetted and updated using national society guidelines and newer research that may not yet have made it into those guidelines.

The information presented at these sites is meant primarily for the medical professional, and assumes the reader has a large amount of basic medical knowledge. Increasingly, they do include a "*For Patients*" section as well.

> ***ICU Confidential Google® That Edition:*** Physicians google information all the time. Really. When we look up a medication or formula we're not sure of, or a rare disease we only remember learning for a test, we use search engines to help get quick answers in real time. The difference is that we generally know what we are looking for, and we can quickly sort through the myriads of information to separate the useless from the useful. As importantly, we know how to interpret and what to do with this information.

J. Family as Advocate, Family as Royal Pain:

In my experience in the ICU, the patient's family members and friends can channel their desire to help in some very particular ways. Some approaches can help if done judiciously, or may possibly negatively impact your stay in the ICU. Let's break these approaches down to a few common family "phenotypes" we encounter, and the recommendations for the best way your family can help you get through this.

i. **The Scientist:** This family member is always ready with a list of questions, lab values, and other test results; they keep track of the vital signs, the IVs, and the ventilator values. They are all about the data, even if they can't necessarily put it into context or make sense of the meaning.

   a. **The Good:** Showing us how invested your family is in your care does reflect well on you and, as much as I hate to admit it, engages us just a little more as well. We expect to be challenged with abnormal test results, so we try just a little bit harder to be prepared to explain minutiae. Although not necessarily contributing to your overall care, this may help you feel more in control, and drives us to make sure your family is better informed.

   b. **The Bad:** While not the most difficult type of family member, this is one we may not go out of our way to seek out (translation: try to avoid). If we happen to see you when that person is not at your bedside, a small twinge of happiness falls over us because this kind of engagement, if done excessively, not only creates a power scenario, but also slows us down. When we have to use all our time to answer questions often having little to do with your actual care, we have less time to provide this actual care.

c. **The Solution:** For us as physicians, we make sure we anticipate these questions and provide answers ahead of time when we give our update. For you as the family member, please be mindful of your physician's time and recognize that the context of these different lab values and other results is as important as the results themselves; don't lose focus of the forest for the trees. Also be mindful that while we would like you to understand the mechanisms behind what's happening to your loved one, we don't always have time to put you through medical school. We do, however, sometimes leave a medical student behind to give you the Cliff's Notes® version (sacrifices must be made; all medical students understand this).

ii. **The Apostle:** Illness is an innately unfair proposition, without justice or logic. Many people may turn to faith to explain what is happening. Sometimes, they believe exclusively in prayer and the power of miracles and positive thinking. They may not seek medical care until their illness is far progressed. In the hospital, they may see the physician's data-driven approach as in conflict with their faith.

a. **The Good:** I personally believe that faith can be an invaluable tool to help you through the most difficult situations. Knowing there is a greater place beyond this life and believing that God's will has a plan allows us to cope and rationalize very difficult situations. Having that backdrop can provide reassurance and comfort. Maintaining hope and positive thinking also play an essential role in your recovery.

b. **The Bad:** Blindly believing in a miraculous recovery precludes even coming to the table to discuss the much more likely alternative (death). This rigid stance may result in hostile relationships with other family members and the medical team. On the other hand, declining potentially life-saving medical procedures because of the belief that the power of faith alone will heal your loved one can also create difficult situations and deny your loved one potentially life saving care.

c. **The Solution:** Having respect for both faith and medical knowledge – these are not mutually exclusive. For us as physicians, this means respecting where you are coming from and meeting you where you are. For you – considering a broader view of faith in the recognition that medical interventions may be viewed as a divine gift and can be accepted in this context. It can also mean that sometimes sparing your loved one these interventions may also be part of God's plan, and that a miracle can happen anytime, *including when we compassionately withdraw life support.* It also means relying on your faith, if that miracle does not happen, to recognize your loved one is at peace in a better place.

iii. **The Invisible Family:** Not everyone has an easy time caring for a loved one in the ICU. Some families may deal with this stress by not showing up. No one in your room, nothing personal on your windowsill, being sent to voicemail when we call with updates or questions.

a. **The Good:** Rounds are faster.

b. **The Bad:** Everything else. Imagine being on a ventilator where you can't speak for yourself and every time we try and find someone to make a decision or give an update, we get silence. Imagine if the only time your medical team hears from your family is when they suddenly call with questions, uninformed accusations, and demands. We obviously take care of our patients the best we can, but not having a partner in the family, especially when the patient cannot communicate, often leads to delays in care and adds uncertainty to an already difficult situation.

c. **The Solution:** We as physicians get that family relationships can be complicated and that folks may have a busy life outside the hospital but this is literally life and death. For us, we can work to identify one individual as the family spokesperson and set expectations at the start. For example, we can schedule a daily phone call with an update and address decisions. For that family spokesperson or medical proxy – please pick up the phone.

iv. **The Demanding Perfectionist:** When nothing is ever good enough and the smallest issues become "completely unacceptable," the likelihood of friction becomes very high. This is the family that chooses to cope with a critical medical situation by blaming the caregivers for anything that's perceived to be out of place. And when nothing is ever good enough and the smallest issues become "completely unacceptable," that can be quite a long list.

a. **The Good:** If you think the squeaky wheel gets all the attention, you're right. Sometimes when things aren't getting done fast enough, yelling fire in a movie theater (ICU) gets all eyes on you. It may not be the right kind of attention, but attention is what you will get (at first).

b. **The Bad:** When even something obviously good is not good enough, we may end up taking your concerns less seriously over time. This breeds frustration and mistrust and can absolutely work against you. It's also hard to lose the reputation of "difficult family." We end up avoiding you, and, more importantly, may spend less time with the patient.

c. **The Solution:** For us, we practice patience and de-escalation. We hear you out, acknowledge valid concerns, and call out misperceptions and unrealistic expectations in a respectful and fact-based way. For you, complaining in this way should be reserved for situations when you truly feel something is off and your loved one isn't getting the attention they need. There is nothing wrong with respectfully calling out things that are not being done right, but please leave room to receive an explanation, and don't forget to acknowledge the things that are being done right.

ICU Confidential: The Prodigal Child Returns: At least once a week in any given ICU, an adult child, usually flying in from far away and having taken no part in their loved one's care, bursts in to read the physicians the riot act. You gave my dad cancer, you mismanaged his stroke, you're trying to kill him by pulling the plug. When this happens we chalk it up to the stress of the situation and your guilt of not being there sooner. It still sucks. Please channel your concerns in a less accusatory way and just don't be that person; we promise to support and explain every detail that you may be concerned about, and to be understanding if approached from a place of respect. And call your mom and dad more often (like now, do it).

v. **The Medically Faithful:** In the bad old days when paternalism was in full swing, the doctor knew everything, and the patient was lucky to be in the presence of such greatness. There was what I consider over-respect and blind faith in the medical system. Some families may still cope by ceding all control of medical care to their physicians.

   a. **The Good:** It definitely makes our lives easier.

   b. **The Bad:** We do want you to take responsibility for the medical decisions involving your loved one. When we make all the medical decisions on our own, we may end up not taking account your loved one's personal goals and choices (since we may not know them), and this may actually lead to less personalized care where we apply a standard solution because we don't have your individual input.

   c. **The Solution:** Let's work together by offering mutual respect that is reinforced by action in both directions. We do want you to have faith in the medical system, but not blind faith and not to the point of excluding yourself from these essential decisions. Please take responsibility for learning about your medical situation (and enlist us to help) so you can make truly informed decisions.

vi. **The Perfect Family, the Perfect Physician:** If this was a feel-good movie, here's how it would be shown in table format:

The Family	The ICU Team
Shows up at the bedside.	Gives time and attention
Asks appropriate questions.	Answers appropriate questions
Is respectful	Is respectful
Mindful of our time	Mindful of your need to know
Invokes faith with eyes wide open	Provides glasses for clarity
Advocates for the patient's wishes, not theirs	Advocates for patient, and their family
Brings donuts	Eats donuts

K. Managing Expectations

It's vital to have reasonable expectations when guiding your care. Understanding what is possible and what is likely can better define your goals and is invaluable in planning for your medical future.

The first reality to embrace is that, unfortunately, patients do not leave the ICU better than they were before whatever happened to get them there. Our interventions only get you well enough so that you don't need to be in the ICU anymore. Being so sick and needing to be on **life support**, heavy duty medications, and the myriads of procedures, can't help but take their toll as well. All along you are getting more deconditioned, having more malnutrition, and more general wear and tear.

For the medical ICU, unless you just had a very sudden trauma or illness, what lands you there is usually preceded by many medical issues. If all goes well, we help you to your feet, but you never get back up quite the same. If you're lucky, you get up enough to walk back towards life as it was before the ICU, with a lot of help and a long road to recovery.

A lot of people look at disease as a battle or a fight, so let's play out that analogy by discussing the general types of ICU patients, and the expectations a patient can have in working towards their recovery.

i. The Chronically Ill Patient:

For most medical ICU patients, they have been slogging it out for a long time, dealing with many medical conditions and their complications. The ICU is a destination after a long, rocky journey which may have included multiple hospital admissions and even prior ICU stays. These patients may have chronic incurable diseases like heart failure and COPD, getting just enough support to eventually leave the hospital, but destined to come back. They may be in and out of a rehabilitation or nursing facilities or barely making it at home.

The ICU is also a repository for end-stage cancer patients dying of their disease and the complications of trying to treat it. Often not ready to transition their fight to comfort, they linger until they ultimately succumb to a complication. The chronically ill patient is the most common type of patient in the MICU.

The goals for recovery must be set in the context of recognizing the toll that chronic medical problems take on the patient's health, and how much worse being critically ill in the ICU can make them. This creates more realistic expectations about the chance of recovery, how long recovery may take, how much rehabilitation may be required, and if ultimately going home is a viable option. It also informs goals of care and end-of-life decisions such as going on a ventilator or accepting other forms of life support.

For some individuals, the ICU will create a road towards recovery through organ transplantation or other form of advanced therapies. Most patients are not candidates for these interventions however (either because their medical problems don't have these solutions, or they are too old or sick to benefit); the ICU will not cure these chronic slowly worsening health conditions, but only help stabilize them (temporarily).

Even patients who are chronically ill, however, may benefit from the evaluation and treatment an acute change in their condition creates. In caring for a worsening of their chronic condition, we have the opportunity to make sure their home medications have been optimized, and that all appropriate treatments have been rendered. We do have situations where your chronic condition was not fully managed and that's why you ended up in the ICU. Finding ways to improve this can be the silver lining in being in the ICU.

ii. The Never Been Sick Patient:

This describes our classic "but he hasn't seen a doctor in 20 years" patient who "suddenly" deteriorates, as well as the person who truly has been very healthy until a dire medical diagnosis renders them in the ICU.

For the former, we may discover multiple undiagnosed conditions like diabetes, heart failure, kidney failure, and the like. They haven't been previously diagnosed or managed because "he hasn't seen a doctor in 20 years."

For the latter, their sudden decline adds another dimension of tragedy and is often incomprehensible to the patient and their family. Examples include a brain aneurysm, major heart attack, aortic dissection, severe head trauma, acute leukemia, and the list goes on.

For patients struggling with the unfamiliarity of being hospitalized let alone in the ICU, please don't be afraid to ask questions and share your concerns. We will always stop and provide the proper orientation and will do our best to guide you through what can be an overwhelming situation.

iii. The Single-Issue Patient:

Fortunately, the rest of you is in pretty in good shape and this adds significantly to your ability to recover. Unfortunately, the degree of the insult can be severe, like a heart attack or a stroke. If that organ starts to bring down the rest, recovery can be long and stressful, but still very likely.

If this describes your situation, know that we will do our best to support you through whatever medical issue brought you to us. Please also remind us that we need to take care of everything else (see the beginning of this chapter) so we don't add any more medical problems to your list.

iv. The Previously Healthy Surgery/Trauma Patient:

Even younger, otherwise healthy patients recovering from trauma or routine surgery are never exactly the same as before the issue that brought them to the ICU, but their chance for recovery is typically very good. Many surgeries are elective (not an emergency), so patients may have time to have their medical conditions optimized and be in other wise reasonably good health prior to the surgery.

In these scenarios, there's a lot of reasons to be hopeful. With time and a lot of hard work, recovery will come. This is the most common patient in the SICU, and they are typically transitioned out of the SICU within a few days.

If this describes you, the best advice is to remain optimistic and to maintain an enthusiastic role in your recovery. This means participating in physical therapy, maintaining your nutrition, and having a positive outlook. This may be difficult if you were previously healthy and are now dealing with pain or new physical limitations but have faith in the body's ability to recover and compensate.

This may not apply for patients that need surgery emergently, or to provide palliation for an otherwise untreatable condition. Many of these patients will struggle due to their advanced medical conditions, poor healing, and complications precluding their recovery. It's important to take this into account when making decisions after trauma or when considering surgery in the first place.

> ***ICU Confidential Hope Me Edition:*** The tenet of never leaving the ICU better than you came in still stands, all other things being equal. When you fully recover from your cancer, you will still be less healthy than before you had cancer. When you recover from your heart attack, you will still be less healthy than before you developed that coronary blockage. However, if there are things about your health you can improve (**modifiable risk factors**), then you can absolutely get better than before you ever got sick!
>
> For example, working on your weight and fitness, quitting smoking, dealing effectively with your stress, and being compliant with your medical regimen are all things that make your health better than it was before. For some patients, getting sick is a wake-up call to change things about their life so they would not get sick again. This can be the best thing that has ever happened to you.

L. The Family Meeting

Communication happens on a continuous basis in the ICU (or should), but there may come a time when everyone sits down to a more formal meeting. This usually means things are not going great, decisions about major interventions and goals of care may need to be made in a timely manner, and more times than not, the patient is no longer well enough to participate.

i. What it is:

While family members are encouraged to be present during rounds and for day-to-day updates, a family meeting is more formally requested during a pivotal point in ICU care, as in when things have really taken a turn for the worse. The meeting puts together essential members of the medical team, the patient (if conscious), and their family (and/or other primary stake holders).

The family meeting is designed to update the family, to answer questions about the current medical conditions, and to inform the medical team of the patient's health care wishes given the situation, in a more formal and documented manner.

ii. Who's in it:

The patient, if they can participate, the medical power of attorney (patient's representative, usually close family or whoever the patient previously designated) and key family and/or friends can be present. On the medical side, the primary team as represented by the attending intensivist with house staff, primary surgeon, and/or primary consultants central to the patient's care (like the oncologist, neurologist, cardiologist, and others) will be in this meeting. It will likely include a nursing representative, the case manager, and possibly a palliative care physician. In cases of high drama (for example, unexpected medical complication or significant friction about your prognosis), a representative from risk management may be there as well.

iii. How it is run:

When everyone is available at the scheduled time, we all meet in the patient's room if they are able to participate. If the patient is unconscious and hooked up to a lot of machines, we can make it a point to find a quiet place with privacy for the patient's family and us, sometimes very hard to do in an ICU.

For my patients and their families, I first introduce myself and all the medical people on the team and make sure to meet every one of the family members (or other health care proxies) present. I typically start the conversation the same way as the code status discussion, by asking the family what their understanding is of the patient's medical condition. I rate their understanding (in a nice way) and proceed to give them a choice to start with their questions, or to allow me to give a synopsis of the patient's conditions first. Once provided, I discuss options moving forward and answer questions along the way.

iv. What is the objective:

It is incredibly important for everyone to be as informed as possible in the patient's medical care. I can't tell you how often we as physicians take vital things for granted, like the patient and their family knowing the degree of illness or assuming the patient's level of understanding about the disease process. We also take for granted that we know the patient's wishes and philosophy on life. The patient and their family may also take for granted the true limits of medical know-how and technology. When we are all well informed, the chance of miscommunication and mistrust becomes much smaller.

Part of being well informed is making sure that all the various subspecialists are talking to each other and providing a comprehensive message. Family meetings are often the place where this can happen.

In a majority of cases, family meetings are called when we think the patient is getting closer to dying and we want everyone to be prepared. So be ready for bad news, and to discuss some important end-of-life decisions. We often re-address **code status** in these situations as priorities begin to shift.

M. Who Do You Ask for Help?

Your primary point of contact at any given time is your ICU nurse and ICU physician. If you have a nursing or physician issue and feel you are not getting anywhere, you can always request the nursing supervisor. Just be patient and respectful and it will be ok. If communication has broken down with your medical team, or you feel like you just can't get your point across, there is another option.

i. Ombudsman, Friend to All:

Every larger hospital has an ombudsman's office that is responsible for investigating concerns about your care. They function like the internal affairs of the hospital. You can call the hospital's main number to be connected or ask for their number from the clerk at the nurse's station.

The ombudsman is tasked with reviewing patient and family concerns and are otherwise independent of your case. They have access to your medical team as well as to the administrators and may serve as your advocate and help bridge any communication issues with your medical team. Keep in mind that your medical team may also contact them to help arbitrate when they feel you or your family are being inappropriate or abusive.

ii. Risk Management:

Usually a lawyer, the risk management professional works to manage the hospital's risk, not yours. They are there to advise staff about medico-legal issues, real or potential. If there's a question about your living will, they may get involved. If there's a medical procedure gone wrong, they may get involved. If you threaten to sue, they definitely get involved. They are there to protect the legal interests of the hospital first and foremost.

iii. Outside Organizations:

There are allies to most any cause. For example, if you need to raise funds for an expensive treatment your insurance doesn't cover, you may consider reaching out directly to the pharmaceutical company or an organization that represents your disease. They may be able to get your treatment subsidized or get you into a clinical trial. They may also point you to specialized care not immediately available where you are.

> ***ICU Confidential Give Peace a Chance Edition:*** When a conflict with a hospital over care cannot be resolved directly, you may think about reaching out to your local news department to plead your case or contacting a political organization that represents your point of view. Please know that getting outsiders involved to try and force your medical team towards doing something they feel is not appropriate will usually cause irreparable damage and rarely works to change the hospital's decisions. You may also lose control of your story when partnering with outside organizations that might use you to champion their cause but will not always put your needs first. If you remain at a stalemate despite best efforts to reach out to your healthcare team, you may consider transferring to another physician or facility more open to your views.
>
> Most importantly, I would strongly encourage you to be honest with your provider and discuss your concerns outright. In my experience, a compromise can usually be found, and differences of opinion bridged. We are all supposed to be on the same team, after all.

Afterword: Putting it All Together

In the ICU, you are thrust into a complex system with many moving parts and many different people. Whether it's your first time getting that sick or your umpteenth visit to the hospital, the fear of not knowing what may be happening with your medical conditions can quickly become overwhelming. We as physicians don't stop and explain the process as well as we should. Couple that with your possibly well-deserved cynicism of the medical system fueled by past experiences (personal or secondary), misinformation, and a context of fear and pain, and you get a perfect scenario for miscommunication and loss of trust.

The solution to this comes from both sides. For us as physicians, it's taking the time to listen to you first, to explain things in an understandable way, to be honest with you about the severity of your conditions, and to match our empathy to our medical skills. For you, it is asking the right questions, having an open mind, and coming to the conversation from a place of mutual respect and at least some degree of trust.

Coming from a more informed place can make all the difference between being anxious and fearful, to being reassured and understanding.

I truly hope that this guide has left you, your family, and your caregivers more informed about the complex world of intensive care. I hope it has empowered you to participate in your medical care, and with the confidence that you are in good and capable hands by explaining what these hands are doing and why. Or it allowed you to recognize that perhaps you are not receiving the best care and informed you of what to do about it.

Either way, information is power, and powerful information is...a superpower.

Appendix

This section contains more detailed information about the various devices, procedures, and medications you are likely to encounter in the ICU. It's here to help demystify the various tests and procedures you may encounter in your own journey, or on your favorite medical TV drama.

While it may contain details that perhaps only a medical student or an engineer may appreciate, this is meant to enhance your understanding of the mechanics of these interventions for those brave souls who are interested.

This section is also the part of this book most prone to becoming obsolete as technology moves forward, so please understand it is in no way meant to be a comprehensive medical textbook.

1 Machines and Things

When you walk into the hospital, you usually have nothing attached (except the emotional strings that bind you). In the emergency department, you usually get a blood pressure cuff, a finger probe showing oximetry and heart rate, and likely some sensors glued to your chest as **EKG** leads transmitting your heart rhythm.

By the time you end up in the ICU, you may have catheters in your urinary orifice (**Foley** catheter), vein (**intravenous** or **central line**), artery (**arterial line**), and stomach (**nasogastric tube**). That's just the price of admission to the VIP section we call the ICU.

Depending on your medical needs, you may end up on a **ventilator** with a plastic tube going down your throat and into your windpipe (**endotracheal tube**), up your rectum (a **rectal tube**), and even more. **Ventilators** and **extra-corporeal membrane oxygenation** (**ECMO**) have already been discussed in detail in Chapter 8: Life Support in the ICU. This appendix describes select other devices and interventions that will be keeping you alive in the ICU, and when you may need them (and when you won't).

Please Note: The following interventions do not represent an exhaustive list (although it may be exhausting reading it). There are new devices coming out some of the time, and a few of these new devices may make our current standard of care obsolete. At the very least, the ones listed below are likely to be improved but not replaced before the next version of this guide. And chances are that if you end up in the ICU, you'll get to know some of them intimately.

A. Basic Monitoring

The ICU monitoring bundle includes a comprehensive package that can look and feel overwhelming. This group of sensors and monitors allows us to track your vital signs frequently and automatically. Tracking some of the more advanced information require invasive sensors and are described later in this appendix.

i. Blood Pressure

Blood pressure (BP) is perhaps the most vital part of your internal body mechanics. It reflects the pressure with which blood is pumped to your vital organs. The top (**systolic**) number represents the maximum pressure that the heart creates in your arteries as it pumps your blood. The bottom (**diastolic**) is the pressure during the relaxation of your heart. Too high a blood pressure and you get direct organ damage (**hypertensive emergency**). Too low and your organs don't get enough blood (this is called **shock**).

Measuring blood pressure consists of a blood pressure cuff around your upper arm that is set to automatically take a reading by inflating the cuff until it cuts off your brachial artery blood supply, and then slowly letting out the air pressure recording when the pulse can be felt. It can be set to take readings at intervals as little as every 30 seconds to every 8 hours.

Sometimes the cuff is placed on your calf, but this gives less reliable measurements. If you have an arterial line (see later in this Appendix), the blood pressure will be taken directly from the catheter and continuously reported. This is more accurate but must be calibrated correctly. If you have a pulmonary artery catheter, the pulmonary artery (blood vessel feeding the lungs) pressure readings may also be reported on the monitor. Other devices estimating heart function also provide on-going readings.

ii. Pulse Oximetry

Oxygen in your blood is carried by a protein called **hemoglobin** that sits in your red blood cell. Think of hemoglobin as a taxi and oxygen as a passenger. The pulse oximeter counts the ratio of taxis that are full (of oxygen) and expresses this as a percentage. This percentage of oxygen in the blood is called the saturation of peripheral oxygen, or **SpO_2**.

The pulse or heart rate is simply a measure of how fast your heart is beating. Both the heart rate and oxygen level can be measured by the pulse oximeter taped around your finger, earlobe, or on your forehead.

The oximeter has two LEDs, one that emits red light and one that emits infrared light. It shines through the finger or ear lobe to a sensor that measures how much of that light passes through (or is reflected back in the case of a forehead sensor).

Hemoglobin that is bound to oxygen absorbs more infrared light versus hemoglobin without oxygen (that absorbs red light). The amount of oxygen circulating in the blood is calculated by comparing how much red and infrared light is absorbed. This is very similar to the pulse oximetry monitor that clips around your finger (the one that everyone rushed to get during Covid).

A reading over 94% is considered normal, and if your SpO2 % is in the 80's or lower, you're in trouble. Keep in mind that you often get an artifactually low number (such as when you are sweating or the sensor loses contact with your skin) so it's important for the provider to check the waveform to confirm the reading.

iii. Continuous Electrocardiogram (ECG or EKG) and Heart Rate

In the ICU you will be attached to several ECG (or EKG in German) wires that continuously report the heart rate and the electrical rhythm in the form of a wave that you can see on the bedside and remote monitor. There is usually a sound that comes with each detected beat. A partial or simplified ECG typically consists of only 3 to 5 leads that are continuously recording (unlike a full or 12 lead ECG). It will pick up most arrhythmias but cannot be relied on to detect all the other cardiac events (like a heart attack) that a full ECG can show (coming up in this appendix).

A full ECG will be performed by the medical team if an active cardiac event is felt to be happening (for example, if you are complaining of chest pain or if the simplified ECG is suggesting an arrhythmia). The simplified bedside ECG is the rhythm you see on TV shows, where the line on the monitor goes flat to indicate the heart has stopped.

iv. Respiratory Rate

Based on your ECG waveforms or a separate band sensor around your chest, your respiratory rate will also be continuously monitored and reported. If you are breathing fast, this may be an indicator of your pain and anxiety levels, but can also suggest a breathing problem that is causing you to need more air. If you are breathing very slowly, you may be oversedated (or meditating). The respiratory rate is prone to error as you move or if it loses connection.

v. Other On-Going Measurements

Your temperature will be measured on a regular basis. An abnormally high temperature (fever) may indicate infection or possibly a drug reaction or other inflammatory condition. A very low temperature can be dangerous, indicating a metabolic, hormonal, or circulatory problem. Temperature can be measured periodically the old fashioned way (a digital thermometer), or continuously with an invasive temperature probe (such as in the bladder, blood vessel, or esophagus).

Your food/fluid intake and urinary and bowel output ("**ins and outs**") will also be recorded. This is especially important if you are in the ICU for a heart or kidney problem. Measurements include any IV medications, as well as any food or drink or gastric tube feeds. Urine is measured based on what comes out of the urinary catheter if you have one, or the urine bottle/pan. Stool is measured as small, medium, or large (or super-sized).

> ***ICU Confidential I'll be Watching You Edition:*** The bedside monitors show vital information about how you are doing, but they are for us and not for you (this is why they are at the head of the bed and you have to look uncomfortably behind you to see them). Please try not to watch these numbers continuously and overreact with every blip or alarm. All these readings are prone to artifact and a momentary misreporting is not an emergency.
>
> The monitors are also being watched and recorded on an outside monitor available to your nurse (and anyone in the hallway!). We wouldn't expect you to perform your own surgery, and we don't expect you to make sense of the data on the monitors. Instead of being glued to the monitor, talk to your family or try to get some sleep. Having said this, if you notice something has been off for a while or the monitor is constantly alarming and no one has come to figure it out, call for the nurse.

B. Catheters for Every Occasion

A catheter is any tube used to facilitate access into a part of your body. This includes the GI tract, the blood stream, the chest cavity, the cerebrospinal space, and every other space inside you. For an explanation of how some common catheters are placed, see Index II: Common Procedures in the ICU. Remember, don't try this at home!

i. Intravenous and Intra-Arterial Catheters:

Medications and fluids can be administered through your gastrointestinal track, skin, lungs, eyes, and, most directly, right into your blood stream. The most basic invasive procedure you will get, likely while still in the ED, is an intravenous (**IV**) catheter. We refer to catheters going into your blood vessels as "lines". These are placed by nurses (they are truly better at it than the doctors), usually in your arm or hand, and usually with a second one for back-up. These hurt only a little and are safe although sometimes they can cause bruising. If left in too long (usually 3 days or more), there is an increased risk of infection and infiltration (torn blood vessel with the medicine going into the soft tissue).

Sometimes, a smaller IV in the hand or arm is not safe for the medications we use. This is because, on rare occasions, IV catheters can puncture and spill contents through a small vein and into the soft tissue, in what is called **extravasation**. If the medication is toxic to soft tissue, damage can occur. Some medications can also cause damage to the smaller veins directly (think **pressors**, see Index III: Medications in the ICU). This is why these types of medications may require larger venous catheters placed directly into larger "central" veins.

a. Central Line

A line going into a larger or central vein is commonly referred to as a **central venous catheter** (**CVC**), "central line", or **triple lumen catheter** (**TLC**), since the most common central catheters have, you guessed it, three skinny channels (lumens) within one catheter. Besides allowing us to more safely use certain medications, central lines also allow for administration of multiple medications at once and can be used to draw blood rather than sticking you over and over again. Another indication for these is when you are being fed through an IV with total parenteral nutrition (TPN).

Central lines are placed in the neck (internal jugular vein), under the clavicle (subclavian vein), or in the groin (femoral vein), allowing direct access to the larger, or central, venous circulation. The neck or chest are usually preferred as they may carry the least risk of infection where bacteria can track down the line, under the skin, and into the blood stream ("**line infection**").

Central lines usually have a lifespan of 7 or so days (less if in the groin, more if you have difficult anatomy and the risk of replacing the line is high). In general, the longer you have a line, the higher the risk of infection. Formation of blood clots can also occur the longer a central line stays in. If a central line is needed longer, other options including a **PICC** (see below) or **tunneled catheter** (where a longer portion of the catheter is placed under the skin).

A central line is not always needed. Even in the ICU, if you have 2 good working IVs, you should be okay. Even pressors can temporarily be run at low dose through a peripheral IV. If you are bleeding (i.e. from your gastrointestinal tract) a large peripheral IV has a bigger lumen than the individual ports of a central line and can handle faster blood transfusions. (On the other hand, if you need rapid infusion of multiple blood products, an **introducer line** has one very large channel that can handle the increased flow.)

If you notice any pain, leaking, bleeding, or swelling around where you have a central line, please let us know right away. Infection, blood clots, and leaking can all be managed easier the sooner we find there is a problem. Also let us know if the dressing has dried blood or is coming off so we can replace this with a fresh one right away. All this is frequently checked by the nurse, but if you notice something wrong, we can get ahead of it even faster.

> ***ICU Confidential the French Edition:*** Catheter diameters are expressed in French (Fr) units, also known as the Charriere (Ch) scale (fancy!). The numbers are calculated by multiplying a catheter's diameter in millimeters (mm) by 3 (for example, a 5 mm catheter would be called 15 Fr). To make it more complicated, peripheral IV catheter diameters are expressed on a gauge (G) scale, with lower G indicating higher diameter (for example, a 22G IV is 0.9 mm wide and a 14G IV is 2.1 mm wide).

b. Dialysis Line:

A special version of a central venous line may be required if you are headed for urgent **hemodialysis**, or kidney **(renal) replacement therapy (RRT)**. The dialysis catheter is larger to accommodate the higher blood flow required in dialysis. When deciding on starting dialysis, needing a dialysis catheter must be taken into account.

A basic dialysis catheter cannot be used for blood draws or medications as it needs to be kept exclusively for the dialysis machine. Some catheters do come with a smaller third channel in the line (Trialysis® catheter) that allows for an extra central access port, including for blood draws.

Like other central lines, there are potential complications with placement of dialysis catheters (bleeding, puncturing the artery when targeting a vein, collapsing a lung), but thankfully these are rare. Ultrasound guidance is the standard of care in placing central lines, and residents and fellows (or physician extenders) usually do them. A chest X-ray is done to confirm placement of central lines placed in the neck or chest.

If a dialysis line is expected to be needed long-term, a **tunneled dialysis catheter** is placed by Surgery or Interventional Radiology. A tunneled catheter is guided (tunneled) in the soft tissue under the skin for part of its length before coming out of the skin. This helps prevent infection and makes it more secure. Versions of this more permanent IV central access also exist for non-dialysis central lines.

c. Arterial Line (A-line):

An A-line is a special type of catheter placed in the arterial system instead of the venous system. This is a thin catheter typically placed in the wrist (**radial artery**), but sometimes in the upper arm, armpit, or even the groin. An arterial line allows for direct and continuous monitoring of the blood pressure through an attached pressure sensor. It also allows for direct sampling of blood from the artery which measures oxygen content and acid-base level (PaO_2 and pH), which is especially important if you are on a ventilator and require frequent arterial blood samples.

You may need an arterial line when your blood pressure is dangerously low and you require pressors that need to be continuously adjusted. There are also devices that help estimate how well your heart is working that can be connected to an arterial line (a FloTrac® or LiDCO® device).

An A-line can hurt a lot more than a venous line since the artery is more sensitive. Placed in the wrist, it can rarely cause a more serious complication by interrupting the blood supply to the hand. This is very rare, and we do a test for alternate circulation before placing the A-line, but it can happen and can lead to gangrene of fingers or the entire hand.

If you have tingling, pain, a change in color, or any discomfort in your hand or arm where there is an arterial line, please let us know right away (actually, let us know if this is happening, arterial line or not).

d. Peripherally Inserted Central Catheter (PICC Line):

A **PICC line** is a very long catheter placed in the forearm that extends into a central vein. Placing a PICC line requires specialized training with using ultrasound and is not done emergently. It is usually placed for longer term IV access needs, including if you need to go home on IV antibiotics for a week or more.

While PICC lines are more comfortable, safer, and have less risk of infection or lung collapse, they require some special expertise and may have a larger possibility of blood clots. As such, if you have a PICC line and the arm is more red or swollen, or if the entry site appears red and/or has drainage, it's important to let us know right away.

e. Pulmonary Artery Catheter (PAC)/Swan Ganz Catheter (SGC):

A pulmonary artery (Swan-Ganz) catheter is an even longer catheter placed through a central vein in your neck. What makes it unique is that it is snaked through the right side of the heart, and into the main circulation of the lungs (into the pulmonary artery). It can be used to draw special blood samples and measure direct pressures in that part of the lung circulation to assist in advanced cardiac care (see Chapter 8: Life Support in the ICU). This is typical in end stage heart failure patients, patients just after their heart surgery, and in patients with severe **pulmonary hypertension** (high blood pressure in the lung circulation).

Like all central lines, it is important that the site they enter the skin remains clean and dry with an intact dressing.

f. Intra-Osseus Catheter:

In a medical emergency, you may have someone coming at you with a small handheld drill. If they are wearing scrubs and a white coat, they are about to put a small but potent intra-osseus (**IO**) catheter directly into your bone, usually your shoulder, leg, or sternum.

An IO catheter is used when an IV line is difficult to obtain, and access is needed right away (like a **Code Blue** situation). The IO catheter allows IV medications to be injected directly into your bone marrow. Because your bone marrow has lots of blood vessels, infused medications quickly make their way into your blood stream. IOs can stay in for 1-2 days, are usually pretty safe, and are not actually as bad as they sound, although they sound pretty bad. Its use is highly dependent on your institution.

ii. Chest Tubes

When there is air in the chest between the lungs and the inner chest wall compressing the lungs, you have a potentially dangerous condition called a **pneumothorax.** This air is usually the result of puncture into the chest through trauma or because of a procedure (like inserting a central line or having a lung biopsy). A pneumothorax can also happen when you are on life support and the ventilator is forced to use high pressures to push air into you and can cause a tear in the lungs. It can also occur spontaneously, especially if you have underlying lung disease like emphysema or chronic obstructive lung disease.

Excess fluid can also get into this space. When it does, the fluid displaces the lung, and you have a **pleural effusion** (liquid in the chest compressing the lungs out of the way). There is always a small amount of fluid in the pleural space to lubricate the movement of the lungs against the chest wall as you breathe in and out, and is constantly being produced and drained by the lymphatic system. If the amount of fluid generated overwhelms the lymphatic collection system, the fluid accumulates in this potential space and displaces the lung. The source can be inflammation (from infection, cancer, and autoimmune disease), or low osmotic pressure (as in low protein states from liver failure, malnutrition, or heart failure), or bleeding from trauma.

Air or fluid can be removed with a single evacuation (**thoracentesis**, see Appendix II: Common Procedures in the ICU) or decompression with a needle (popular in medical TV shows and movies [Angry Max was apparently an EMT before the apocalypse]).

When continuous evacuation is needed (especially for air), a catheter called a **chest tube** can be placed. This can be a more rigid surgical chest tube for thicker fluid (brutal), or a thinner flexible tube (genteel and preferred) that can be placed using a needle introducer. The thin flexible type of tube is sometimes called a **pig-tail catheter.** No real pig's tails are involved — the name comes from its curly shape (like a pig's tail) so it can collect more fluid from multiple ports and has less of a chance of being dislodged.

Chest tubes are usually connected to a tall plastic box on the floor that collects the fluid and is connected to a suction tube going to one of the vacuum nozzles sticking out of the wall by the head of the bed. Please don't knock this over. If you do, don't just place it back upright. Tell the nurse so they can fix it correctly (you can blame your clumsy cousin who just left).

There are also versions of chest tubes (PleurX®, Aspira®, and others) that can be tunneled under the skin like the long-term dialysis catheters. The outer part of the catheter has a one way valve so air can't go inside the chest, and is coiled and placed under a dressing on the skin. A vacuum bulb can be connected to the catheter hub every couple of days to drain the fluid from the chest. By allowing intermittent drainage, this type of catheter can serve as a bridge until the underlying cause can be fixed (after which the catheter is removed). This is also offered when someone needs repeated evacuation of fluid for palliation, like in advanced heart failure or cancer, and can be managed at home including through hospice. These tunneled chest tubes are not typically done acutely in the ICU, but may be offered to help get you home afterwards.

iii. Gastric Tubes

When a patient is confused, somnolent, or having other issues with swallowing, a **nasogastric tube** provides a temporary solution. This soft catheter is inserted through your nose and down into the stomach. It allows medications and nutrition to be delivered directly into the stomach when you can't safely swallow on your own.

Placing these catheters is unpleasant (for you and for us), and they can be incorrectly inserted into the airway/trachea instead of the stomach. A chest X-ray is routinely done to confirm proper positioning so tube feeds aren't sent into the lungs.

There are a few versions of these gastric tubes. The larger one (**Salem Sump**® or **Levin**®) gets clogged less often but is less comfortable, and the smaller one (**Dobhoff**®) is easier on the patient and can go beyond the stomach but gets clogged more often and has a higher chance of being placed incorrectly in the trachea. A **Corpak**® feeding tube is another option that is somewhat more rigid but allows extra monitoring during insertion to allow it to pass just beyond the stomach.

The feeding tube is usually taped to your nose, but a nasal bridle can also be used to securely anchor it with a clever magnetic probe that guides it through the nostril to the back of the nose and brings it out the other nostril to be tied together.

If you are intubated, the gastric tube usually goes through your mouth (**orogastric**) right next to the breathing (endotracheal) tube. Hopefully, you are sedated enough and don't notice.

It's important to note that only medications that can be crushed can go through a gastric tube. Some medications are specially coated and need to be swallowed whole to work, especially certain long-acting formulations.

iv. Percutaneous Endoscopic Gastrostomy (PEG) Tubes

A feeding tube placed directly through the abdomen and stomach wall is called a PEG tube. PEG tubes are usually placed through the skin by a gastroenterologist or surgeon. A tube with a camera at the tip goes down your throat and into your stomach for guidance (**endoscopy**). Once inserted through the abdominal wall, the PEG tube is held in place with a balloon at its tip inside your stomach. In complicated anatomic situations, this may have to be done surgically.

PEG tubes are meant for long term use when you cannot swallow reliably on your own. Scenarios include having a severe stroke or another condition where you are not able to wake up enough to eat or swallow reliably. Having a stroke or surgery that affects your swallowing muscles also counts. Being on a ventilator long term also usually necessitates a PEG tube, although there are certain situations where you are ventilated through a tracheostomy and are awake and interactive enough to eat.

PEG tubes are safer and generally more comfortable for long term use than orogastric and nasogastric tubes. As mentioned above, these often go with tracheostomies in getting you ready for long term rehab or chronic care.

v. Urinary Catheter

Also known as a **Foley® catheter**, a urinary catheter is a soft catheter that is inserted through the urethra and into the bladder.

There is a balloon surrounding the inner end which is inflated once the catheter is inserted to hold it in place inside the urinary bladder. A Foley catheter prevents incontinence and allows accurate recording of how much urine you generate. It also bypasses most partial obstructions (think enlarged prostate). Urinary catheters can also be used to indirectly measure the intraabdominal pressure in situations where this can be dangerously high (like in abdominal infections, bleeding, fluid buildup [ascites], and so on).

Aside from the discomfort and a constant feeling that you have to urinate, there is a risk of infection, with bacteria tracking up the catheter and into the bladder and beyond. Also, confused patients sometimes pull these out, inflated balloon and all (yes, you read that right). There are external versions of urinary catheters for men (condom catheters) and women (adhesive options) that may be more comfortable and safer but often leak.

vi. Other Tubes in All the Right Places

There are additional specialty catheters depending on the situation. For example, patients with strokes or bleeding in the brain may need an **intracranial pressure monitor** and/or drain (a catheter that sits in the brain through a small hole in the skull). Examples include intracranial (inside the skull) or intraventricular (inside the ventrical or fluid collection in the center of the brain) catheters.

Sometimes, a catheter is placed through the front of the chest into the sack around your heart (**pericardial sac**) when there's a fluid buildup compressing your heart function (**pericardial effusion**). Sometimes catheters are placed in the gallbladder or in an abscess to drain and decompress it (think liver or gut), or into the kidneys if a kidney stone is blocking urine from getting out (**nephrostomy tube**). Then there are the rectal tubes for people with non-stop diarrhea. There really is a catheter for every opening or cavity!

Depending on the type of catheter, it may be put in by different specialists: for example, an interventional radiologist (like for an inflamed gallbladder or abscess), or neurosurgeon (intracranial or intraventricular catheters).

> ***ICU Confidential You Look Young to be a Doctor Edition:*** You may be wondering if the most senior person on the team should be placing a catheter into the sickest patient. The truth of the matter is that

an attending physician may not have personally placed a catheter in years (!), especially if they oversee a large academic team. Typically, "see one do one teach one" applies, and there's a long list of residents and fellows very happy to put these in. And they get really good at them. The senior members of the team may supervise, or if the procedure is deemed particularly difficult, they may be the ones placing the catheter directly (for example, if you are very obese or your blood vessels have a lot of scarring).

Please don't feel you are getting experimented on if the most senior person on the team isn't the one placing your catheter – that may actually be a good thing. Having said this, you are well within your rights to ask any of your physicians or physician extenders how many procedures they've done, and (diplomatically) suggest that you would feel better with a more senior member of the team. If you have a very junior member of the team, they'll always be supervised at the bedside by more senior staff.

ICU Confidential Bonus Content: All major procedures and surgeries, unless in an emergency, require **informed consent.** This is where the proceduralist explains the intervention, risks and benefits, and alternatives, if any. This step is unfortunately all too often rushed or skimmed over, and sometimes even just performed by the nurse with *"Sign here if you want to live,"* in an Austrian accent, of course.

The nurse or physician should never be placing a complicated form in front of you and telling you to sign it without an appropriate explanation. I always take the extra few minutes to do this right. It informs you as a patient and makes sure this is what you want. And it protects us because complications do happen (even with our always perfect technique!), and then we can say we informed you that these may happen because we did.

ICU Confidential Director's Cut Edition: It is vital that any catheter be taken out as soon as it is no longer essential. The longer these catheters stay, the higher the chance of infections and other complications. In truth, they sometimes get overlooked or left in because it's easier (think a nice neat rectal tube versus having to do clean up on aisle 6 every 2 hours). The best ICUs assess the need for these catheters daily and have systems in place to ensure they are removed as soon as possible. Don't be afraid to ask if you still need that catheter.

C. Respiratory Devices

Breathing does two specific things: it provides oxygen and removes carbon dioxide. This requires a complex respiratory system of mechanics (muscles, bones and airways) and membranes (lungs and alveoli) that have to work together to keep you alive.

Below, you will find a number of interventions that can compensate for issues in the respiratory system, starting with how we increase oxygen, to how we take over the mechanics of breathing. Please note that ventilators and extra-corporeal membrane oxygenation (ECMO) are described separately in Chapter 8: Life Support in the ICU.

i. Oxygen, High Flow, and Nebulizers

Oxygen is absolutely essential for life. Fortunately, our lungs are pretty good at extracting it from the air we breathe and have plenty of reserve (which allows us to run fast and lift heavy things). When you lose enough of this reserve and need more than regular air has to offer, we have a number of ways of increasing the amount of oxygen going to your lungs.

a. Nasal Cannula

The nasal oxygen cannula is the basic plastic nose tubing everyone seems to get as soon as they get a hospital bed whether or not it's needed. This cannula is meant to deliver additional oxygen compared to regular air in your room ("room air" is 21% oxygen, 78% nitrogen, and 1% other/flatus).

The amount of additional oxygen is determined by how many liters of pure oxygen flow through the cannula per minute. Each liter adds about 3% to the oxygen content to the air you are breathing, but the higher it goes the less reliable this calculation.

Your blood oxygen level is estimated from the **pulse oximeter** on your finger or ear lobe (95% and up is normal, below 88/89% you need extra oxygen) or directly from your blood through an arterial blood gas (or if you just look in distress and are struggling for more air).

Once you're past 5 or 6 liters by nasal cannula (about 40% oxygen at best), it's usually time to move on to another type of oxygen delivery system. Nasal cannula systems can be seen outside the hospital for patients with chronic lung diseases, as well as for anti-smoking TV ads.

b. Oxygen Masks

There are different types of oxygen masks designed to deliver from 28% oxygen all the way to 100%. A venturi or **Venti-mask**® can be set to approximate percentages up to about 60%. A **non-rebreather mask** usually means you're in trouble as it's delivering up to 100% oxygen. These are the masks with the see-through plastic jock-strap shape and a reservoir bag sometimes attached beneath it. It encloses the nose and mouth, thereby limiting how much ambient (21%) air you get with every breath. Nowadays, these types of masks have been all but replaced by high flow oxygen systems.

c. High-Flow Oxygen Systems

When your oxygen level needs more than a little support, we turn to a system where a very high flow of air mixed with extra oxygen comes through a more robust cannula that typically fits snugly into or immediately surrounding your nares. A high-flow oxygen apparatus allows us to set a very high flow of air as well as the percentage of oxygen in that air.

High-flow oxygen systems form a partial "flow" seal of sorts and makes it a bit easier to breathe since air is being delivered so forcefully. For example, if a nasal cannula delivers 5 liters of oxygen per minute, this type of system flows up to 50 or 60 liters of air per minute. The incoming air can be regulated to consist of up to 100% oxygen. It can also be humidified and heated so you can better withstand that level of air flow. At the time of this writing, this is the oxygenation method of choice when you have very low oxygen levels (**hypoxia**).

There is a milder form of this therapy that can deliver oxygen at moderate rates, usually up to 10 liters of air per minute with up to 50% oxygen, termed **mid-flow oxygen**.

d. Nebulizers

Medications can be mixed with a small amount of sterile salt water (**saline**) and be aerosolized to create a fine mist. You can breathe this in through a mouthpiece or a mask, thereby delivering medication directly into the lungs. The nebulizer does not form a seal and a lot of the medication escapes, especially as you breathe out. Note that no special technique is needed to use a nebulizer. This means that it can be used at home for asthma or COPD therapy. Special medications that help open the airways, provide anti-inflammatory effects, and even some antibiotics can be administered this way, including in the ICU. A special adapter allows nebulized medications to be delivered through the ventilator as well.

ii. Noninvasive Ventilation (BPAP/NIPPV)

When extra oxygen and higher flow rates are not enough, you get to have a positive pressure experience. Positive pressure refers to the pushing action of oxygenated air through a tightly sealed mask (think fighter pilot's mask).

An external air pump pushes oxygen through the mask into your lungs through your mouth and throat. This piece of equipment is commonly referred to as a **Bilevel Positive Airway Pressure** (**BPAP**) machine. A BPAP can deliver mandatory breaths if you stop breathing (when in spontaneous timed, or –**ST mode**) and can show how much air it delivers at a given pressure. There are fancier versions that are basically ventilators attached to you through a mask instead of an internal (**endotracheal**) tube. All these ventilation machines are types of Non-Invasive Positive Pressure Ventilation, or **NIPPV**.

Chronic obstructive pulmonary disease (**COPD**) and **congestive heart failure** (**CHF**) exacerbations are the most common scenarios where NIPPV can be lifesaving. This has been shown to save more lives than going directly to a ventilator, so it is usually worth a try if you're not too far gone. Other situations like muscle failure (think neurologic issues like Myasthenia Gravis or Guillan-Barré syndrome) also warrant its use. Even though it's uncomfortable, you are usually pretty air hungry by the time you need this so you'll take all the help you can get.

Remember, BPAP or NIPPV is meant to be a *temporary support* while the underlying problem is being improved upon – think peeing out (diuresing) or dialyizing the excess fluid in a heart failure exacerbation or steroids and antibiotics to open up the airways in COPD exacerbations, or while a ventilator makes its way to your room. An exit strategy here is essential since you can't eat, drink, swallow medications, or talk while this is on, and it's pretty tight so skin breakdown (especially the bridge of your nose) is almost guaranteed.

NIPPV may be familiar to those with sleep apnea. **CPAP (continuous positive airway pressure)** or BPAP therapy commonly used for obstructive sleep apnea can be thought of as a type of NIPPV. In sleep apnea, CPAP and BPAP are used to keep an overly relaxed upper airway (back of the throat) from collapsing while you sleep when you are otherwise doing okay. In the ICU, NIPPV is used at much higher pressures and for a very different purpose.

> ***ICU Confidential No NIPPV for You Edition:*** While NIPPV is often a bridge to being on a ventilator, it can save you from that very special experience, but only in certain situations. If you are confused or somnolent (very sleepy) for whatever reason, if you have a lot of phlegm with pneumonia, or if you have a lung collapse, NIPPV can actually be harmful, and a ventilator is more appropriate if in line with your goals of care. NIPPV can also be used to help get you off the ventilator faster, where you are extubated to NIPPV — kind of like an in-between step before you are breathing completely on your own. This type of support must be used judiciously, and temporarily. It is generally acceptable even if you have a **Do Not Intubate / Do Not Resuscitate** (**DNI/DNR**) order, although like all interventions, you have the right to decline it.

> ***ICU Confidential Prequel Edition:*** Non-invasive ventilation should technically only be used if you are awake/arousable and can take off the mask if you need to. Imagine throwing up and being too weak to take off the mask. NIPPV will blow those chunks right into your lungs. I can't tell you how many times I've seen somnolent patients in restraints while on BPAP in the regular hospital ward. Except in very select circumstances where there is direct observation like in the ICU, and with no other options, the risk benefit equation of using NIPPV on barely conscious patients needs careful consideration.

iii. Ventilators:

When you are so sick that you can't breathe on your own at all, you may be put on a ventilator, the fundamental life support intervention in an ICU.

Ventilators can provide complete support for your respiratory system, breathing completely for you (pushing air into your lungs via a fancy air compressor) and delivering oxygen in the most efficient way (something the less invasive systems above cannot do). A ventilator can also be set to deliver partial support for when you are able to participate. A ventilator in the ICU is the same technology you get in a more controlled setting when undergoing anesthesia for elective surgery.

You can read much more about these devices in Chapters 8: Life Support in the ICU and in Appendix II.

iv. Tracheostomy Tubes

When you are unable to use your upper airway (nose, mouth, throat) to breathe, a much shorter, curved plastic tube can be inserted directly into your windpipe (**trachea**). In the ICU, this typically happens when you've been on a ventilator with an endotracheal tube for too long, and there's no immediate proverbial light at the end of the tunnel.

When you first get intubated, you have a longer tube that goes through your mouth, down your throat and into your main airway. It's connected to the ventilator which helps you breathe and is called an **endotracheal tube (ETT)**. After about 2 weeks of this, the risk of pneumonia from the endotracheal tube starts to increase significantly. The risk of soft tissue breakdown and bleeding also goes up.

At this point, unless you're almost ready to be extubated and just need another day or two where the tube can be removed, and you are breathing on your own, a tracheostomy is recommended. Sometimes, it's done earlier if you have problems with your upper airway anatomy (like tongue or throat cancer). Rarely, it's done as a surgical emergency (like during a severe allergic reaction with severe swelling [**angioedema**], or inability to secure an airway any other way during attempted intubation).

The tracheostomy is a surgical procedure that can be done by a surgeon in the operating room, or sometimes right at the bedside if the anatomy is straightforward. Some intensivists, especially in the Surgical ICU, have training in this.

> ***ICU Confidential Packaged to Go Edition:*** In most ICUs, tracheostomy is the green light for transfer to a long-term facility that can handle a ventilator. Because of the inherent danger of endotracheal tube displacement, clogging, or other malfunction, most long-term acute care hospitals (**LTACHs**, for rehabilitation and recovery) or chronic ventilator facilities (slow death) don't take ventilated patients unless they are ventilated through a tracheostomy tube. Don't delay the tracheostomy because of this – if you are not stable in other ways, you cannot go to a long-term facility anyway. Also, the danger of delaying tracheostomy for non-medical reasons can lead to infection and death. Just recognize that having a tracheostomy tube typically means you may be packing for your next destination. If you need a tracheostomy for long-term care, you usually also get a surgically implanted feeding tube (PEG, see above). More on this in Chapter 11: What Happens After the ICU.

D. Radiology Tests and Procedures

The field of radiology has grown tremendously since the birth of the humble X-ray. Using different modalities like magnetic fields (MRIs), sound waves (ultrasounds), and nuclear tracers, we now have many incredible tools to help us diagnose serious medical conditions so we can hopefully fix them.

i. X-Rays and CT Scans

Getting a chest X-ray (**CXR**) in the ICU is almost as common as getting your labs done. Typically, everyone on a ventilator gets a CXR once a day to check the positioning of the endotracheal tube and what the chest looks like. The same applies if you have a pulmonary artery catheter or other active cardiac support devices. Abdominal X-rays (kidney, ureter, and bladder X-ray, or **KUB**) are performed to look at problems in the gut, as well as to check the positioning of a feeding tube. X-rays are done to look at joints and limbs as well, to make sure there's no dislocation or fracture. These all carry very little radiation (we are told), and it's not uncommon for you to have dozens of these before you're ready to check out of the ICU. Most of these can be done in your ICU room.

A **computer-aided tomography** (**CT**) scan is a bunch of X-rays taken at different angles that the computer processes and puts in a very detailed 3-D format. Looking at a CT is like looking inside you without having to cut you open. These scans are done on much larger machines and required a trip to the radiology department. You are transferred from the hospital bed to the CT table and pass through the center of a large donut-shaped machine containing the X-ray emitters and sensors. CTs are essential in evaluating stroke or bleeding in the brain, pneumonias, intra-abdominal abnormalities, tumors, and much more. They can be done with injection of **IV contrast** (dye) and/or oral contrast for abdominal CTs depending on what we are looking for. A special contrast version called a CT pulmonary angiogram is also used to look for blood clots in the lung (**pulmonary emboli**).

CTs emit a lot more radiation than regular X-rays but are still relatively safe to do. However, since radiation exposure is cumulative, having too many CTs can carry long-term radiation risk.

> ***ICU Confidential Field Trip Edition:*** It could be that a CT (or another radiology test that requires transport) is medically needed, but you are too sick to go. Leaving the relative control and safety of the ICU, going through hundreds of feet of hallway, often requiring an elevator, and then being moved from your hospital bed to the scanner and back may seem like a nice change of scenery. But if your blood pressure is dangerously low and needing multiple pressors, or you are on a ventilator with very high settings, this field trip can be your last. There's nothing like hearing "Code Blue in CT #4" — the CT scanner is a heck of a place to try to do CPR. In summary, if you technically need a CT but your doctor (or nurse) isn't letting you go, there's a very good reason, and a bad sign.

ii. Ultrasound

Ultrasound is one of our best friends in the ICU. Its many wonderful uses range from checking for blood clots in the legs (**lower extremity doppler**) or your overall heart function (**echocardiogram**, described separately), to using it extensively for line placement, blood volume assessment, finding abnormalities in the lungs or abdomen, and more. In fact, we now often do our morning rounds with an ultrasound machine in tow, checking many of these things in real time. It's harmless (sound waves!) and provides a lot of useful information when done correctly.

iii. MRIs and MRAs

Magnetic resonance imaging/magnetic resonance angiograms (MRIs/MRAs) are an imaging technology which highlights in detail the state of solid organs like brain, bone, muscle, and heart. This technology isn't used well for lungs – they are not solid enough. MRIs can also be done with special contrast (dyes) depending on the indication.

MRIs are rarely emergencies in the ICU but can be essential in evaluating stroke and other brain and spinal cord pathology. Different types of MRIs are done for many types of indications. A special MRI called **magnetic resonance cholangiopancreatography (MRCP)** looks specifically at your gallbladder and biliary system to evaluate for gallstones and infection. An MRI of the heart is also done to look for **amyloidosis**, a rare infiltrative disease that can affect heart muscles.

These magnetic scans take a lot more dedication and time (very narrow bed tunnel, loud, claustrophobic) and can pull metal right out of your body. For all types of MRIs, your body must be metal free (or have "safe" metal not affected by a magnet) and relatively stable, and for hospital patients, it's usually done when the outpatient time slots are off (like late at night).

> ***ICU Confidential MRI Edition:*** The magnet of an MRI machine is always on. This requires special "magnet-safe" versions of the equipment that usually accompanies you from the ICU, including special ventilators, IV pumps, and the like.

> ***ICU Confidential "Don't Code in the MRI" Edition:*** Aside from the magnet always being on, it can take up to 10 minutes to power down an MRI machine and get you to a safe (Zone IV) space to fully perform resuscitation. If you code in the machine, staff may not be able to get to you for that length of time to fully try to revive you; we can only treat you with thoughts and prayers.

iv. Ventilation and Perfusion (V/Q) Scan

This nuclear medicine scan is done to rule out smaller blood clots in the lung, including when you are allergic to IV contrast or kidney failure and cannot get a **CT angiogram**.

A V/Q scan works by using two (very low dose) radioactive tracers, one in the air you breathe during the test, and the other injected into the blood stream. It uses a special **gamma camera** to show where these tracers go to create images of the air in the breath you are holding and the other in the blood stream. If the images match, you are not likely to have a blood clot. If the blood tracer is missing in an area where the air tracer is present, it is likely because a blood clot is preventing blood flow to that area.

A V/Q scan can show smaller and more chronic blood clots a little better but does not show the lungs well, like a CT would. It can also be less accurate if you have other things going on in the lungs (like pneumonia or scar tissue). V/Q scans are also done for outpatients with chronic embolic disease. They are performed in the nuclear medicine part of the Radiology department.

v. HIDA Scans

A **hepatobiliary iminodiacetic acid** (HIDA) scan is not only a mouthful, but also a nuclear medicine scan designed to assess problems of the liver, gallbladder, and bile duct. It involves injecting a radioactive tracer (very low dose) into a vein and performing a scan with a gamma camera. This shows how and where bile is flowing to help identify any blockages, inflammation, or leaks. HIDA scans are used when ultrasound or CT alone are not enough to make a diagnosis. It requires a field trip to Radiology and an injection, followed by another trip two to four hours later (after the tracer has time to fully flow through the biliary system).

vi. PET Scans

Positron emission tomography (PET) scans involve injecting the body with radiolabeled sugar, allowing it to circulate, and then performing the scan to see where in the body this sugar accumulates. Collections of cells that are "hungrier" than their neighbors, like rapidly dividing cancer cells or infection-fighting cells needing more energy, pick up and concentrate this sugar.

PET scans are typically done in an outpatient setting for staging to see if a cancer has spread, or for cancer surveillance to see if a cancer has come back. On occasion, it may be used in the ICU environment to help guide care. It is a full body scan and comes with a full body (lower quality) CT for overlay mapping. We often take advantage of the CT portion and help you avoid getting a separate CT to find out what's going on. The PET/CT takes 3 plus hours.

vii. Angiograms

An angiogram involves direct injection of contrast material in the artery or vein of whatever body part you want to map the circulation of while taking continuous X-rays or a specifically timed CT scan. For example, it can be used to look at brain circulation when trying to identify bleeding or an aneurysm. It can also be used to assess the circulation of a limb, the gut, or the lungs, and is performed by Interventional Radiologists in their procedure areas.

E. Dialysis and Plasma Exchangers/Plasmapheresis

Dialysis, or **renal replacement therapy** (**RRT**), in the ICU is similar conceptually to dialysis in the outpatient setting. People live for many years devoting 3-4 hours to a dialysis center 3 days a week. Some people even do it at home, including nightly through what's called **peritoneal dialysis** (or even hemodialysis). Starting dialysis in the ICU, however, is considered a type of life support as it is usually part of the multi-organ failure cascade that predicts a poor outcome.

The dialysis machine works through a large catheter in your vein (**dialysis line**, see section B above) or a surgically placed **arterio-venous fistula** in your arm (common in long-term use for outpatients). It removes blood from your vein and filters it in a variety of ways before returning it back into your bloodstream (usually this uses the same catheter with two channels inside it). The opening for the blood return tube is positioned downstream of the collection tube (you don't want to get this wrong).

This machine is designed to take the place of the kidneys when they fail. Sometimes, this technology is used to remove certain toxins from the blood, or to help control high potassium or blood acid levels, or to remove excess fluid from the body quickly. Rarely it is used to remove some overdosed drugs/medications.

Dialysis can also be used to remove certain immune complexes in cases of acute auto-immune disease, exchanging the part of your blood that contains your immune proteins (plasma). This is called **plasma exchange** or **plasmapheresis**.

There are different forms of dialysis depending on how quickly you can tolerate the flow. The standard is called intermittent hemodialysis (**IHD**) and takes 3-4 hours (same as outside the hospital). Sometimes dialysis must be run more slowly but continuously because your blood pressure is too low and cannot tolerate IHD. To get the same effect, it must be run continuously and not just for 3-4 hours (24/7 until the crisis resolves). This includes **sustained low-efficiency dialysis (SLED)**, **continuous veno-venous hemodialysis (CVVHD)**, and another even slower type called **ultrafiltration** or **UF** (*go Gators!*).

The kidneys may be recoverable, or the dialysis you start in the ICU may become a chronic outpatient therapy. In many ways starting dialysis in the ICU is a more difficult decision than having time to prepare for it in the nephrologist's office. In the ICU, needing dialysis, and especially CVVHD, is not a good sign. On the contrary, coming off CVVHD because you are tolerating normal dialysis, and coming off dialysis altogether, are definitely good signs!

F. Neurologic Monitoring

If you are in the ICU for a neurologic issue such as a stroke or central nervous system infection, special monitoring becomes essential to your recovery. Aside from very careful neurologic exams looking for subtle physical and mental changes ("**neuro checks**"), there are several devices that help us figure out how you are really doing.

i. Electroencephalograms (EEG)

If you are admitted with any situation where seizures are a possibility, you get a nice person (maybe they're not nice, I don't know) that comes and attaches multiple electrodes across your scalp. The technician places these electrodes via an adhesive and does not pierce the skin. The electrodes send a continuous recording of the electrical activity of your brain from which seizures or other general neurologic conditions can be detected (including brain activity slowing or **encephalopathy**).

ii. Intracranial Pressure (ICP) Monitors

If you have a lot of swelling in the brain and things are getting tight inside the skull, your neurosurgeon may elect to put a small device directly through a hole in the skull to monitor the pressure inside;

this is called an Intracranial Pressure or ICP monitor. Versions of these can act as drains as well. This helps decompress the skull cavity to help avoid damaging the brain. If the intra-cranial pressure gets too high and medications aren't able to control it, cutting the skull open may be necessary. This is usually no big deal. Just kidding, this is a really big deal.

G. Cardiac Devices

From the simple and invaluable ECG to the partial heart function replacement left ventricular assist device, below you will find explanations of the most common heart monitoring and interventions seen in the ICU.

i. Electrocardiograms

This is a classic (invented in 1902) and still very reliable technology that allows us to diagnose arrhythmias, heart attacks, sometimes electrolyte disturbances, and even drug toxicities. As described in section A, the **ECG** or **EKG** is where we put a bunch of small adhesives on your chest, arms, and legs and attach sensor wires that are tuned to pick up the electrical activity of your heart.

A standard or complete ECG has 12 leads using 10 sensors (electrodes) placed on the arms, legs, and multiple points along your chest. While more comprehensive, it only provides a 10 second snapshot of your heart rhythm.

Interpreting an ECG is a skill in and of itself, but there can be very obvious clues as to what's going on. In fact, it is still the fastest and most reliable test for acute heart attacks and arrhythmias. It is completely harmless except for the bonus waxing when taking off the adhesives.

ii. Echocardiograms

While technically an ultrasound (as mentioned above), these are unique enough to get a section of their own. **Trans-thoracic echocardiograms (TTEs)** are a way to easily evaluate how strongly the heart is pumping, how well the heart valves are working, and if there's fluid around the heart. It gives us an idea of lung circulation as well. All this is done with some lube jelly and a probe on the surface of your chest. If you have a lot of swelling (or are particularly fluffy), the pictures don't turn out as well.

If we are concerned about a hole in the heart where the blood goes from one side to the other skipping the lungs (cardiac shunt), air bubble type contrast can be used (TTE with **agitated saline** or contrast).

There is also a special type of echocardiogram where we look from the inside of your esophagus called a **trans-esophageal echocardiogram** (**TEE**). This requires sedation because a relatively thick tube that is the ultrasound probe is stuck down your throat and lodged midway down your esophagus. The view from there gives a much better look at the back side of the heart, especially the heart valves. This may be recommended if there is concern for an infection seeding a heart valve, a condition called **endocarditis**.

iii. Intra-Aortic Balloon Pumps, Impellas™, Aortix™, Tandem Heart, Ventricular Assist Devices and More

When your heart function drops to dangerously low levels where it can no longer pump blood well enough through your body, you generally go into multi-organ failure and die. We refer to this as heart failure and it can happen after a heart attack, a heart valve issue, or through the natural progression of other chronic heart disease. You can get help from medications, but when they are not enough, you may benefit from some mechanical assistance.

Depending on the situation, the **intra-aortic balloon pump** (**IABP**) is generally the first mechanical support step when medications alone are not enough. An IABP is inserted through the artery by way of a catheter and sits in the aorta close to where the left ventricle (the powerhouse of the heart) pushes oxygenated blood to the rest of the body. After the heart squeezes, it relaxes to refill for the next push. This is called **diastole** and is where the balloon pump inflates to give an extra mechanical push making sure the coronaries are well perfused, and the blood continues to push forward to your organs.

If an IABP is not enough, a miniature **ventricular assist device** (**VAD**), most commonly an Impella® or Aortix®, is used. It is also placed by winding a catheter up the aorta and into the left ventricle where it helps pump blood and is a higher level of support than a balloon pump. These come in different variations, and the larger more powerful (and riskier) versions require surgical monitoring.

It's important to realize these devices are a bridge to something else (think days not weeks). They are designed to give the heart time to recover from a temporary shock, time to get to a definitive surgery, time to transition to a chronic IV medication, or to heart transplantation.

The traditional left VAD (**LVAD**) is a larger more potent version of the miniature ones. It completely takes over the pumping of the left side of the heart (a version can sometimes be used for the right side of the heart as well [**RVAD**]). This can be portable and a destination therapy if you can't get a transplant, but may also be used as a (longer) bridge to transplant.

A Tandem Heart® is another catheter-based support device. It is placed through the large vein to the right side of the heart but requires a puncture inside the top part of the heart (atrial septum), takes longer to put in, and is not meant to be used for an extended period. For more information about advance cardiac support, see Chapter 8, Life Support in the ICU.

> ***ICU Confidential Location Location Location Edition:*** These advanced cardiac assist devices are typically placed through a groin artery and snaked up to the aorta or the heart. This means you have to stay flat, sometimes for days. Try eating, stretching, or moving your bowels when you are flat in bed! A more difficult but better for mobility technique involves placing these devices through the underarm or upper body. This can only be done with some devices and may be more technically difficult and possibly riskier, but it means you can sit up, move your legs, and more. Ask your cardiologist or surgeon if this may be appropriate.

H. Restraints

While not exactly procedures, restraints represent an intervention that's very important to know about. It may seem strange to talk about tying someone down who isn't under arrest or into some alternative recreation (no judgement), but you can absolutely be dangerous due to being very confused and disoriented in the ICU.

Whether you are confused because of the illness that brought you to the ICU, confused because of the interventions in the ICU, or confused because you've lost all sense of day and night, you can become violent to yourself and us. You may have some dementia or other underlying health issues predisposing you to this as well.

In the ICU, it's not uncommon to be connected to multiple IV lines, catheters from which you pee and poop, and lots of monitor-related wires (blood pressure cuff, oxygen finger sensor, ECG leads, and so forth). You may have fresh surgical staples or be hooked up to a dialysis machine or a ventilator, all things that shouldn't be removed unexpectedly or by force. This is where restraints can help.

Restraints come in different physical forms, from mittens on hands to wrists being tied down to the bed rails to only allow for limited movement. 4-point restraints include the ankles as well. All these restraints require well-documented reasons for their use, and safeguards for prompt removal as soon as it is safe to do so.

Chemical restraints can refer to sedative medications used to keep you safe, especially when you are on a ventilator. A few types of protocols are used to help guide your nurse as to how sedated you need to be, such as the **Richmond Agitation-Sedation Scale (RAAS)**.

As the preferred alternative, redirection through conversation and gentle physical reminders with someone by your bedside can often go a long way in avoiding extra sedation or physical restraints.

> ***ICU Confidential You're Hired Edition:*** There are standard protocols for sedation while on a ventilator, each allowing for personalization depending on how you respond. For situations where you can get away with minimal or no drugs or bindings, you may want your family and friends to take shifts keeping you comfortable. Being presented with a familiar face and voice when you are scared and confused can really go a long way in calming you down. We absolutely love this kind of family participation and support (as opposed to just coming and complaining).
>
> As an alternative for when your family can't be there, we may have a **sitter** for you. This is an entry level (poorly paid) staff member that's required to sit by your bedside, hopefully talk to you, and catch your hand before it grasps some important tube and yanks it out. Often, sitters can be seen on their phone or simply sleeping, but at least it's something (and technically they are sitting). Translation for families: please be there if you can.

ICU Confidential, Push and Pull Edition: While our goal is always to minimize sedation in the ICU, this is often a push and pull scenario. The nurses mostly have control of how much sedative you are getting, and when to give additional "as needed" sedatives. This is based on specific scales that take into account your pain level, vital signs, level of agitation, etc., but some of it is very subjective. It's no surprise that the use of sedation medications goes up overnight. This is in part to keep you safe, certainly, but you have to wonder if staying quiet overnight means our job is also quieter (this never happens). Of course, the last thing we want is self-extubation (you pulling out your own breathing tube) in the middle of the night when less personnel are around to save you, but we also don't want you to be zonked in the morning when we are ready to try and get you extubated in a controlled setting.

2 Common Procedures in the ICU

This section outlines the patient's experience for procedures commonly performed in the ICU, in case you or your loved one are about to have one done.

My hope is that in reading these descriptions you can be better prepared for what actually happens during these procedures, as well as be able to raise more well-informed concerns with your medical team. It may even help you recognize what care is needed after. As always, please, don't try any of these on yourself, or on anyone else.

> ***ICU Confidential Before We Start Edition:*** Please note that for all these procedures there are a number of things that should be done consistently and properly. The first is providing proper education and obtaining **informed consent**. The next is making sure the operator has performed **hand hygiene** and is wearing the appropriate **personal protection equipment** (**PPE**) like a surgical mask, surgical hat, sterile gloves, and sterile smock if needed. This is non-negotiable and you are encouraged to call out the medical team if this is not being done (maybe in non-confrontational way, like noting "It must drive you crazy to wash your hands 30 times a day").

A. Central Line and Arterial Line Placement

As discussed in Appendix I, Machines and Things, a **central venous catheter** or central line is a large catheter designed to go into one of the main (central) veins. An arterial catheter is a catheter that goes into an artery to directly measure blood pressure and allow for collection of **arterial blood gases**.

i. Central Line

Common sites for this catheter include the internal jugular vein in the side of the neck, the subclavian vein under the clavicle, and the femoral vein in the groin. Each site has its advantages and disadvantages, and the right site is based on a number of factors including your anatomy, prior complications, and physician experience.

For example, the neck (internal jugular) and subclavian (under the clavicle) sites are generally preferred as they are less likely to cause infections, but these sites have a higher risk of puncturing and collapsing the lung. The clavicle site is cleaner and more comfortable to live with but is not easily compressible if you bleed. The groin site may be more prone to infections but is generally easier to put in and compressible in case of bleeding. It also cannot collapse the lung (if it does, call 1-800-easy-money).

The procedure starts as all procedures do, with informed consent where we explain why we're recommending a central line, what bad things can happen, and what the alternatives are, if any. We specifically discuss bleeding, lung collapse, introduction of infection, pain, and **air embolus** (rare). Once you shrug and sign on the bottom line, we are ready to go.

First, we generally evaluate the prospective sites (neck, clavicle, groin if needed) to make sure there's no skin infection, other cuts, or other barriers to success. We then use an ultrasound to help visualize the vein. If we are targeting the neck or clavicle, we put you in the **Trendelenburg** position where the legs are elevated above the head. This position puts more blood into the vein and makes for a larger target. It also helps limit the possibility of an air embolus traveling to the brain.

The operator sanitizes their hands and then puts on sterile garb (gloves, gown, hat, mask, looking good). The area is cleaned and then you get a large sterile drape that covers everything outside that 4–5-inch area where the catheter will go. Of note, the sterile sheet usually covers your face, so be prepared for this. You typically have an oxygen cannula running under the drape or are on a ventilator, so you will be okay.

The area is cleaned again. An ultrasound probe with a sterile cover is used to visualize the vein and confirm the proper approach. The transducer jelly for the ultrasound will feel cold and wet. A small amount of lidocaine is then injected first just under the skin, and then deeper into the tissues, causing a sharp and burning sensation. Once the area is comfortably numb, the operator will place a large caliber needle with a syringe with the stopper being pulled back to create a small vacuum as she advances it deeper towards the vein.

Ultrasound is being used continuously at this stage to track the advancing needle in relation to the large blood vessel it's targeting. Once the needle pierces the vein, dark blood briskly fills the vacuumed syringe (and indicates success). The operator then removes the syringe while keeping the needle in place and feeds a flexible metal guidewire through the needle. The needle is then removed from the body, leaving only the guidewire, one end in the vein and the other sticking out of you. Ultrasound is used to confirm the guidewire is in the vessel and going the correct way (towards the heart). You may be feeling some pressure and a little wet from the hopefully scant blood that came out of the needle, but no pain per se.

A scalpel is used to nick the anesthetized skin where the guidewire enters to give room for the semi-rigid dilator and flexible silicone/plastic catheter to be inserted over the guidewire. A special tool called a dilator is passed along the wire to open the tissues so the thicker catheter can be inserted. If the central line is a hemodialysis line, multiple dilators are used to create a larger opening. The operator infuses the catheter with sterile saline and then feeds it into the vein over the guidewire. When the guidewire comes out of the other end of the catheter, she removes the guidewire so only the catheter remains.

We confirm blood return and then suture the hub of the catheter to your skin so all our hard work doesn't go to waste when you accidentally try to yank it out during the night. A special dressing finishes the job, and the sterile drapes are removed. We give each other a knowing nod. A chest X-ray is used to confirm placement of the jugular and subclavian catheters.

ii. Arterial line

Arterial lines are usually placed in the radial artery in the wrist. When you have poor circulation, an artery in the mid, upper, or under arm is used. In cases where the anatomy is very difficult, we use the femoral artery in the groin. Arterial lines take more experience and placing them is also risky, with the most common complications being bleeding and triggering an arterial blood clot. In the wrist, occluding the artery can cut off the blood supply to the hand and cause gangrene if not corrected quickly. We are required to check for collateral circulation that can prevent this, (called the **Allen Test**), but the test is not fool-proof.

The operator sanitizes their hands, puts on protective gear, and obtains consent informing you of the dangers listed above. After cleaning the skin around the target, a smaller sterile drape is used to cover the surrounding area. Sometimes, the operator uses a small amount of anesthetic, but this injection can also hurt as the artery itself cannot be anesthetized. Ultrasound guidance is helpful, but just feeling for the artery can be enough. A needle is used to access the artery until a flash of blood return is seen.

If we are just collecting a sample, the needle is withdrawn, and you're done. This blood sample is called an **arterial blood gas** and provides valuable information about the oxygen and acid-base content in your blood. If a catheter is to be left in, it usually follows a small guidewire introduced through the needle. When the guidewire passes through the needle, the needle is removed, and the catheter is passed along the guidewire. The guidewire is removed and discarded, and the catheter is left in while the hub is secured with a suture and special dressing. Sometimes a wrist splint is used to keep the catheter from losing signal due to positioning.

> ***ICU Confidential Do I Really Need This Catheter Edition:*** Avoiding a catheter unless it is truly needed is the best way to avoid complications. On the other hand, very few physicians are looking to take any extra risks, so if a catheter is being recommended, it's likely to be necessary. To prevent complications like infection and blood clots, catheters should be removed as soon as they are no longer essential.

> ***ICU Confidential 2, Origin Story Edition:*** When you consent to medical procedures and interventions like special medications that require a central line or dialysis, you will also need to consent to the access catheters necessary to run them. It's a package deal, so you must factor that into your decisions.

> ***ICU Confidential 3, Return of ICU Confidential Edition:*** Many larger medical centers will have a vascular access team. Their job is not only to get IVs in difficult access patients but also offer **mid-lines** (a cross between an **IV** and a **PICC** line, see Appendix I for details about IVs and PICC lines). These teams may not be available after hours but may be worth the wait. If your line is not an emergency and can wait

for this team, it may be worth bringing this up with your physician. You may end up with a safer catheter.

B. Intubation

When you are in respiratory distress (or heading there), are somnolent, or are being put to sleep for surgery, you will be going on a ventilator. Intubation is the process of getting you on that ventilator.

Intubation involves giving you significant sedation and sometimes paralytics, putting a special tool called a **laryngoscope** with a camera equivalent through your mouth, and guiding a semi-rigid plastic tube down your throat and through the vocal cords. This tube is then connected to the ventilator, and you are now on **life support**. As noted, several paths can lead you to require intubation, all involving the fact that you can no longer reliably breathe on your own.

We typically use a protocol called **rapid sequence intubation** (**RSI**) given the typically urgent nature of ICU (and ED) intubations. This is the preferred, standard-of-care method for securing an emergency airway using a sedative and paralytic to rapidly induce unconsciousness and paralysis.

We obtain consent, when possible, as this is often done emergently, like during a **Code Blue**. We tell you basically that there is a tangible chance you could die, but also that you may feel like you can't breathe, feel pain and choking, and that you won't be able to talk or eat once you are attached to a ventilator. We talk about the alternative, usually a very high risk of death, possibly **non-invasive ventilation** (**NIPPV**), and/or transition to comfort care. Provided you or your loved one say yes, we take a deep breath and get everything, and everyone, ready – this is truly a team effort.

We position ourselves behind you at the head of the bed. We make sure we have all our equipment – the video laryngoscope (usually, although old-school direct visualization laryngoscopy is still done), the **endotracheal tube** (**ETT**), a semi-rigid stylet in that tube to give it shape, a suction catheter, a ventilation bag with oxygen going through it, an air filled syringe to fill the ETT cuff that will help it stay in place once inserted, and a CO2 detector to help confirm the tube is in the right place. Joining us is a nurse, a respiratory therapist, sometimes an additional physician to assist, and a cup of

Cuban coffee. We make sure the respiratory therapist has back-up equipment (plans B & C), has the ventilator set up and on stand-by, and is ready to help with an extra pair of skilled hands.

The nurse checks your IV and prepares the sedative and usually a paralytic medication under our direction. We position you towards the head of the bed, elevate the bed to a comfortable position for us, sometimes put a rolled-up towel under the small of your back to make your airway more prominent, and briefly check your airway (say ah) and your chin to neck distance. Then we down the Cuban coffee and we're ready to go.

We give the order for the nurse to first inject the sedative (etomidate, propofol, versed, fentanyl, ketamine – lots of choices, see Appendix III, Medications in the ICU). We wait the appropriate minute or so to make sure you're unconscious while providing oxygen and extra breaths through an external ventilation mask and then inject the paralytic (best not to get the order mixed up). The paralytic helps us open your mouth and position you correctly and without resistance. We check that your jaw is lax, extend your neck (**sniffing position**), and get ready to insert the video (or direct) laryngoscope, a rigid L-shaped tool with a handle that lets us move your tongue out of the way and lift the tissues in your throat. This tool provides a video feed to a small monitor at the base of the laryngoscope or a video monitor on a pole next to you (or a direct but more difficult view).

We position the laryngoscope down your throat pushing the tongue out of the way and lift to see the most beautiful site in the world — the gates of pulmonary heaven known as the vocal cords. We suction out any material that may be obscuring our view and pass the ETT through the vocal cords while withdrawing the stylet.

If we are having difficulty with your anatomy, we can resort to placing a temporary airway device called **a laryngeal mask airway (LMA)**. This can be placed blindly through the back of your throat and creates a seal around your larynx with an inflatable cuff. It is less dependable but can provide precious minutes before more help arrives. We can also use a **bronchoscope** (a longer flexible tube with a camera and direction control) or pass a special semi-rigid plastic rod called a **bougie** through the cords and pass the endotracheal tube over it (these are plans B through D).

When we believe we are in good position, we inflate the cuff on the ETT, connect the ETT to the ventilation bag, and give a few breaths while we check the CO2 detector. A team member listens to the lungs and the stomach area while we give a few breaths and hopefully hear them going into both lungs and not the stomach. The ETT gets connected to the ventilator and the happy juice (sedation) starts flowing in a continuous stream through your IV so you don't wake up to feel the choking sensation or pain. We thank the team for a job well done and give ourselves a mental high five.

ICU Confidential No Guarantees Edition: Whether it's because of a massive **aspiration** (vomiting into the upper airways and the lungs) or severe bleeding in the airway, losing the ability to see the airway anatomy is the operator's worst-case scenario. There is no way to reliably intubate someone by "feel". All the specialized tools we use to help visualize the airway depend on being able to see with the camera, and the camera doesn't have wiper blades.

Old school direct visualization can also be difficult if all you're seeing is red. Sometimes the only option is to perform an emergency **cricothyroidotomy** where we access the windpipe directly through the neck (**tracheostomy**). This takes special tools, time, and experience. If we can't suction the obstructing material or dilute it out with saline irrigation, or get an airway directly through the throat, you will likely die.

The overall success rate for intubations (by the second attempt) is highest for dedicated critical care teams, and still has an expected failure rate of up to 6%.

C. Thoracentesis and Paracentesis

There are two main body cavities that can accumulate a lot of fluid quickly or over a long period of time - the chest cavity and the abdomen. When the amount of fluid starts to cause problems, and it cannot be treated with medications, it may need to be drained. This procedure is called thoracentesis when removing fluid from the chest, and paracentesis when removing fluid from the abdomen.

i. Thoracentesis

The chest cavity houses the heart, pipes and wiring (esophagus, lymphatic system, blood vessels, and nerves), and two compressible balloons called lungs (actually, two lobes on the left and three on the right, connected at the stem). Between the lungs and the inner chest wall is a potential space called the pleural space.

There is always a small amount of fluid in the pleural space to lubricate the movement of the lungs against the chest wall as you breathe in and out, but when it builds up due to infection, cancer, or bleeding, among many other reasons, you get what is called a **pleural effusion**. If this gets very large and causes breathing issues, your condition warrants physical evacuation of this fluid with a procedure called a thoracentesis, and goes as follows:

After obtaining consent which apprises you of the most common complications like collapsing a lung (**pneumothorax**), chest wall pain, bleeding, and introducing infection, we sanitize hands and don proper attire. You'll usually be placed in a sitting position at the side of the bed hunched slightly over to rest on one of those moveable bedside tables. The operator identifies the safest pocket of fluid using ultrasound (our favorite), marks it with a sophisticated medical tool (a pen), and then proceeds to clean the area and apply the sterile drape.

We numb the skin with lidocaine, passing the needle deeper into the chest until we get some return of liquid from the syringe. You may feel a pinch (medical-speak for a sharp pain like when you're being stabbed in the chest with a needle). We withdraw this needle, nick the skin with the scalpel at that site, and advance a much larger needle wearing a soft catheter. The large needle has a syringe which we keep at negative pressure and when fluid flows into it, we know we're deep enough.

At this point, the needle stays steady while the soft catheter is advanced over it into the chest cavity. The needle is retracted, and the end of the catheter is left in the cavity while we attach the tubing to the outside end. We then remove as much fluid as is safe and send it to the laboratory for analysis. When you start to feel chest pressure and an insatiable need to cough, we know we've removed enough.

We ask you to hum while we take the catheter out. The humming prevents you from taking a deep breath and potentially sucking air through the hole left by the catheter, causing a collapsed lung due to external air. We do a spot check with ultrasound. We then shake hands all around and tell you what a good job you've done (by just sitting there). A chest X-ray is routinely performed to make sure there is no procedure-related lung collapse.

Of note, if we expect that you will continue to need drainage over the ensuing days, we can leave the catheter inside the chest and connect it to a drainage box. The catheter is then called a **chest** or **thoracostomy tube**, and the whole procedure is similar.

Another variation of this procedure is used to evacuate trapped air in the chest (and outside the lung, called a **pneumothorax**), except the catheter is usually left in and is also connected to a suction box to continue draining the air.

ii. Paracentesis

Fluid can also accumulate in your abdomen surrounding the bowels, the liver, and the rest of the abdominal organs. That fluid may be there from liver failure with low protein in the blood, and can also come from abdominal infections, cancer, bleeding, or complications of peritoneal dialysis. While the abdominal contents are mostly non-compressible, the soft tissues enveloping the abdomen can expand quite a bit. This potential space between the abdominal organs and the abdominal wall can fill up with fluid and cause significant discomfort.

In addition to pain, the ducts going from the kidneys to the urinary bladder (**ureters**) and the kidneys themselves can be compressed by the pressure generated from this fluid. In extreme cases, this can damage the kidneys through obstruction.

When it is determined that the fluid should be removed, it is done as follows:

We obtain consent which apprises you of the most common complications like bleeding, nicking the bowel or other abdominal organs, pain, introducing infection, and low blood pressure (**hypotension**). Once you agree, the operator sanitizes their hands and puts on proper garb. They will first use ultrasound to identify a good site (pocket) to put in the needle. They then clean the area, put on a sterile drape, and chit chat about your favorite sports team while we get everything ready.

We re-clean and then numb the area using a needle with lidocaine down to the point that we get fluid back. We may use a more rigid, blunt metal catheter that surrounds the needle, minimizing the risk of internal bleeding. The catheter tip is positioned in the abdomen while we're draining the fluid after the needle is withdrawn. A sample of the fluid is sent for analysis and culture. There's tubing connecting the needle hub to a wall vacuum or similar device that will help the fluid come out – we can remove 5 to 10 liters at a time. Easiest way to lose weight quickly.

Sometimes the above procedures are done by Interventional Radiology. This is more typical in the subacute or outpatient setting.

D. Lumbar Punctures

Taking a sample of cerebrospinal fluid surrounding your spine is sometimes necessary to check for a central nervous system infection or for less common neurologic diseases (like Guillain-Barré syndrome). A lumbar puncture is similar to placing an epidural catheter during childbirth, except the goal is usually to just take a sample without leaving a catheter in the spinal canal.

First, we obtain consent when we talk to you about pain and possible complications: bleeding into your spinal canal, partial paralysis (!), and introducing infection. Headaches and back pain can persist post-procedure. Provided you still say yes, you are then placed in a fetal position with knees raised and back hunched over as much as possible to open the spaces between the vertebrae. Alternatively, you can be sitting and hunched over while leaning on one of those movable tray tables like you did for your thoracentesis.

We sanitize our hands, put on proper attire, and clean the area between the vertebrae in your lower back below where the spinal cord turns into millions of smaller fibers. A sterile drape is placed to cover the surrounding area, and the skin is re-cleaned and anesthetized. A separate needle is advanced between the vertebrae and into your spinal canal, and a small amount of cerebrospinal fluid is withdrawn. A device is usually used to measure the opening pressure as well.

Lumbar punctures can be done by the intensivist, neurologist, or interventional radiologist (if the anatomy is very difficult requiring real-time imaging).

E. Bronchoscopy

By now, you've likely realized that –oscopy means a scope in some part of the body. With bronchoscopy, we are going into the airways (bronchi) of the lungs. The bronchoscope has an appropriately small camera sensor at the tip and openings for suctioning and for passing small instruments like brushes or micro forceps for obtaining samples. We control the direction of the tip of the scope as well, allowing a measure of navigation.

The bronchoscope is passed through the mouth or nose, down your throat, and into the windpipe (trachea) and larger airways (bronchi). Bronchoscopy may be done to clear out heavy secretion of pus and mucus or aspirated materials, get samples directly from the lower airways to analyze for infection, look around for cancer, or even take out a misguided peanut (this does happen, especially in kids).

After obtaining consent where we talk to you about coughing, choking, having a sore throat, bleeding, introducing infection, and respiratory failure, and you say yes, we sanitize hands, put on proper PPE, get you into position and have you breathe in some nebulized lidocaine. We then give you some happy drugs (versed, fentanyl, sometimes propofol), and when you are in twilight sleep, we put in a special mouthpiece which protects both your very expensive teeth and our even more expensive bronchoscope.

We insert the bronchoscope through the mouth and track down the throat to visualize the vocal cords, spray them with lidocaine through the bronchoscope, and then proceed through them into the windpipe (trachea). Like the branches of an upside-down tree dividing from the trunk (the trachea is the trunk), the airways divide into the left and right main stem bronchi and then further still. Like the branches of a tree, the further out you go the more the bronchi taper and the thinner they become. This limits how far the main part of the bronchoscope can go.

We have several ways to get beyond where the bronchoscope can physically pass. For example, we can spray sterile water into the farthest reaches of the airways through the bronchoscope, and then suction the water mixed with the airways contents back to send for analysis (**bronchoalveolar lavage**). We can also pass very small brushes, a wire basket, and very small forceps to take bread-crumb sized pieces of whatever needs sampling.

If you are already on a ventilator, we pass the bronchoscope through the endotracheal tube. This is much simpler since you are already sedated and we have full control of the airway. If you have a tracheostomy, we use that opening to directly access the trachea. It's much easier, but we charge the same.

Bronchoscopy gets very fancy very fast. We have robotic bronchoscopy to sample lung nodules way out in the periphery of the lung, ultrasound to biopsy lymph nodes, argon plasma coagulation to zap open tumor laden airways and stop bleeding, balloon dilatation, airway stenting and more. In fact, there is now a subspecialty within the subspecialty where your **pulmonologist** (lung doctor) takes on more formal training (interventional pulmonary fellowship) to be able to do all this. These advanced bronchoscopy techniques require specialized equipment and can be done in the ICU under certain circumstances. Sometimes, complex bronchoscopy procedures require ICU care afterwards since the patient may still be on a ventilator.

F. Endoscopy, Colonoscopy, PEG Tubes, and FEES

Whether it's to look for bleeding in your gastrointestinal (GI) track or to look for a source of obstruction in your gut (think cancer, ulcers, infections, and more), a fiber optic cable can be passed through the mouth and into the esophagus and stomach in the case of endoscopy, or through the anus and into the large intestine in the case of colonoscopy. Like the bronchoscope, an endoscope has the equivalent of a camera at the end of it and has channels through which suctioning can be performed and fluid and medication can be injected. A separate channel allows fine tools like forceps and loops to be passed through.

i. Endoscopy

When we are concerned that you have an upper GI bleed (bleeding coming from the esophagus, stomach, or duodenum) or an abnormality like a mass on imaging, we talk to you about doing an upper endoscopy. After obtaining consent when we discuss the risks of bleeding, vomiting, pain, sedation, and perforation of the digestive tract, and you still say yes, we proceed to give you happy drugs to put you into twilight sleep. We wash hands and don proper attire, ask Siri to put on Coldplay and spray numbing medicine into the back of your throat.

The endoscope is passed along the tongue to the back of the throat and beyond, bypassing the vocal cord area, down the esophagus, and into the stomach. A video is transmitted in real time to the operator, and biopsies and brush samples of different sorts can be obtained. Therapies like lasers, banding, biopsies, and injections, as well as other interventions, can be done to stop bleeding, fill in ulcers, and close off abnormal blood vessels (**varices**).

Endoscopy is usually done with moderate sedation while you breathe on your own but can be done (even easier) if you are already on a ventilator and deeply sedated. Endoscopy is performed by the gastroenterologist.

ii. Colonoscopy

Like an endoscope, the colonoscope is a fiberoptic steerable cable with channels that allow for different interventions. It's also a camera without a windshield wiper so the fuller the lower gut is with blood or stool, the less you can see through the colonoscope. Sedation is used, but typically not to the point of general anesthesia. The procedure (and interventions) is similar to endoscopy, with location making the difference. Like an endoscopy, a colonoscopy can be done in the ICU room (if you're too sick to travel) or in the GI suite. A gastroenterologist performs the procedure, and an anesthesiologist typically controls your sedation and well-being.

Colonoscopy in the ICU setting is done urgently to visualize cancers, bleeding, obstruction and other abnormalities, and it allows us to take biopsies, apply different techniques to stop bleeding, and offer additional interventions. It can identify situations where surgery may need to take place as well.

In the outpatient setting, colonoscopies save lots of lives with colon cancer screening. If you're fifty (or forty-five) or older, get it done!

ICU Confidential Catch 22 Edition: Your GI consultant is often stuck between you being too sick to perform an endoscopy or colonoscopy, asking for stabilization in the form of blood transfusions, blood pressure control, intubation for airway control, correction of blood thinners and the like, and not being sick enough to need an emergent procedure. Sometimes the reason you need an endoscopy is to fix whatever's making you too sick to get an endoscopy in the first place, so now you're stuck. Have an honest conversation with the proceduralist and make them commit to the procedure or give you definitive parameters of what would allow them to proceed.

ICU Confidential Extra Innings Edition: If your procedure turns out to not be emergent, you are often told to get it done after you go home (as an **outpatient**). The healthier you are, the less risky the procedure, so the reason often given is that you need to be healthy enough to leave the hospital first. The truth is usually one of logistics, resources, and, yes, insurance. If you've ever tried to schedule a screening colonoscopy, for example, you know you often typically wait weeks to get insurance approval and an actual available date and time. In the hospital, you expect it to happen the same day or the next. This puts a lot of strain on all the staff and resources that are required, often at the expense of outpatient availability for someone else.

In addition, you have the financial question. When you are hospitalized, the hospital is usually paid a pre-negotiated lump sum based on your diagnosis (bundled into a single **diagnosis-related group** [**DRG**] re-imbursement). Depending on insurance, they may not pay for the procedure separately if you get it as an inpatient. This applies to many procedures that are usually done for non-hospitalized patients. You hate to think that influences the hospital's decision, but when money is involved, your convenience becomes much less of a priority.

iii. Percutaneous Endoscopic Gastrostomy (PEG) Tubes

Endoscopy is also used by gastroenterologists or surgeons to place a catheter called a percutaneous endoscopic gastrostomy tube. This tube goes through your abdomen directly into your stomach to provide feeding and medications when you can no longer swallow on your own.

The procedure includes marking the insertion site in your upper abdomen guided by imaging and the light from the endoscope from inside the stomach (if you ever shined a flashlight through your finger, you know what I mean). The area is sterilized, and a small incision is made through which the tube is passed through the skin and into the stomach. The endoscope confirms that the tube is properly positioned. The PEG tube has a balloon towards its tip which is inflated once it is in the stomach to hold it in place. PEG tubes are done under conscious sedation similar to endoscopies, and local anesthesia.

iv. Fiberoptic Endoscopic Evaluation of Swallowing (FEES) and Video Fluoroscopic Swallow Exam (VFSE)/ Barium Swallow

Conditions affecting swallowing include stroke, surgery or trauma to the throat, and being on a ventilator for a long time. Chronic conditions like advanced dementia, failure to thrive and neurologic muscle wasting (like amyotrophic lateral sclerosis or ALS) can also impair your ability to swallow. Swallowing not only applies to food and drink, but also to saliva and other secretions. Aspirating these contents into your lungs causes inflammation and damage (and even pneumonia).

a. FEES:

Performed by a **Speech-Language Pathologist** or **Speech Therapist**, the fiberoptic endoscopic evaluation of swallowing is performed to assess your ability to swallow and make sure you are not aspirating into your lungs. A thin, flexible fiberoptic cable is passed through the nose down your throat with the equivalent of a camera at the tip, similar to the other "oscopies" described above. Different consistencies of food are then given for you to swallow, and their transition is directly observed to see if anything goes down the windpipe instead of the esophagus.

b. VFSE/Barium Swallow:

Alternatively, a video fluoroscopic swallow study or modified barium swallow exam can be done. This is where a special X-ray film is taken while you swallow food of different consistencies. The barium is mixed with the food and can easily be seen on the X-ray allowing the radiologist to tell if all of it is going down into your stomach, or your lungs. It also outlines the shape of the throat and esophagus, showing major abnormalities that may need additional testing.

G. Cardiac Catheterizations

Non-invasive testing like an ECG, echocardiogram, calcium score CT, or a stress test is very useful in identifying **coronary artery disease** (**CAD**: blockages in the arteries supplying the heart muscle with blood). Those tests also sometimes come back normal even when you are having significant symptoms that we suspect are heart related. This is when cardiac catheterization ("cath") becomes necessary. Cardiac caths allows accurate diagnosis of CAD and also treatment. They are also useful in identifying a condition called **pulmonary artery hypertension** by directly measuring the pressures from the right side of the heart.

Caths are usually done as an outpatient procedure when things are stable. When you are hospitalized with an acute event and things are getting critical, we get it done urgently/emergently. Depending on which side of the heart you're looking at – left for arteries/coronaries, right for pulmonary circulation pressures, the procedure goes something like this:

i. Left Heart Catheterization

The left heart catheterization allows your cardiologist to visualize the anatomy of the **coronary arteries,** the all-important arteries feeding the heart itself. It also allows us to visualize the function of the left ventricle, the powerhouse of the heart responsible for pushing blood into the rest of the body. We can also see the left atrium, the set-up chamber accepting the oxygenated blood from the lung circulation and pushing it into the left ventricle, and the valve (mitral valve) between them.

As for other procedures, we obtain consent by telling you about possible bleeding, infection, perforation of the blood vessel, heart attack, arrhythmias, stroke, blood clots, aneurysms, anesthesia risk, and exposure to radiation. While all these things are possible, they happen rarely, and this procedure can be absolutely lifesaving.

The cardiologist determines the best approach, typically using the femoral artery in the groin or the radial artery in the wrist.

After performing hand hygiene and putting on appropriate PPE, the cardiologist starts by accessing the artery with a needle and replacing it with a sheath (a large IV through which a catheter can be passed), the cardiologist inserts the catheter into the artery and snakes it back towards the heart.

They can see where it's going by using continuous X-rays (**fluoroscopy**). They also use IV contrast injected through the catheter at specific points of the procedure. By seeing how and at what rate the IV contrast moves through your coronary arteries (the blood vessels that provide blood supply to the heart muscle) on fluoroscopy, they can detect blockages. They can also open these blockages by inflating a very small balloon at the tip of the catheter (**angioplasty**) and deploy a **cardiac stent** through the catheter to keep the blood vessel open.

Once the procedure is complete and the catheter withdrawn, a pressure device is placed where the artery was accessed (like in the groin) for a number of hours to minimize any bleeding or bruising. You usually must lie flat for that time. If the procedure is high risk or you've experienced a complication, you will usually come to the ICU to be carefully monitored.

ii. Right Heart Catheterization

While left heart catheterization is by far the most common since coronary artery disease remains the number one killer of American adults (thank you, French fries, cigarettes, and scrolling instead of strolling), right heart catheterization (**RHC**) is still very important. It is used to evaluate the fluid balance in the lungs in advanced heart failure, and high blood pressure in the lung circulation (**pulmonary hypertension**) by directly measuring these pressures through the catheter. This is often used to figure out if the symptoms are coming from the heart or the lungs, and what types of advanced heart therapies may be most effective. RHC also allows a pulmonary artery catheter to be placed that can then guide pulmonary hypertension and advanced heart failure therapy in the ICU.

Right heart catheterization starts at the groin or neck vein, a low-pressure system with fewer bleeding complications. Using on-going X-rays (**fluoroscopy**) as a guide, the catheter snakes through the right side of the heart (right atrium to the right ventricle). From there, the catheter goes to the pulmonary artery, the main blood vessel feeding the lungs oxygen depleted blood. A pressure transducer allows direct measurement of this circulation along with a number of other parameters that we use to figure out that the problem is in the heart *and* the lungs.

H. Wound Care

The most important part of wound care is not getting a pressure-induced wound in the first place. This can be accomplished by strictly following turning protocols (every 2 hours), getting you out of bed as soon as you are able, making sure you have the right mattress and support, and keeping up with your nutritional needs. Good nursing care makes wounds manageable and even preventable.

Unfortunately, if you have a stroke and can't move, if you're cancer has reduced you to skin and bones, if you have severe malnutrition while still being overweight, and/or if you're on a chronic ventilator, pressure ulcers around your backside (at the tailbone) are still very likely to develop. Called **sacral decubitus ulcers**, they are staged at different levels depending on how deep and how wide they go. The higher the stage, the worse the wound, up to "unstageable." If the bone is exposed, infection of the bone can set in (**osteomyelitis**), a dangerous condition requiring prolonged antibiotic treatment.

Wound care professionals are nurses and physicians with specialized training and experience, and strong stomachs. Depending on the location and characteristics of the wound, they make recommendations in terms of what medications to apply, the dressings to cover them, if a **wound vacuum** is required, and if they need surgical debridement to remove unhealthy/dead tissue and accelerate healing. If surgery is needed, a plastic surgeon or general surgeon is usually called in to perform the task, typically right at the bedside.

While this section applies to pressure induced wounds or bed sores, surgical and trauma related wounds also need meticulous care so that infection can be prevented and healing can occur.

> ***ICU Confidential Pain in the Sacrum Edition:*** Sacral (tailbone) ulcers are a common quality marker for nursing care. Long term ventilator facilities and nursing homes are notorious for breeding these kinds of ulcers due to lack of nursing support, nutrition, proper wound care, and, of course, the condition of patients they deal with.

> You can use this as a quality marker when looking for a facility, so be sure to request the data – they are required to report it to the Centers for Medicare and Medicaid Services and the state health department in most states. Having said this, we often see the worst sacral ulcers coming from severely impaired patients cared for at home where the family was not equipped to perform the necessary preventive care.

> ***ICU Confidential, a 2nd Movement Edition:*** Wounds near the butt are sometimes difficult to heal as they get infected by contact with stool. If things get particularly bad, a **diverting colostomy** is sometimes performed where your colon is diverted to come out your lower abdominal wall so you poop into a pouch far away from the wound (into a **colostomy bag**). Once the wound heals, the colon can be reconnected so you can poop as nature intended.

I. Parenteral Nutrition

Feeding you directly into your blood stream is called parenteral nutrition. When done through a peripheral intravenous (**IV**) line, we call this Peripheral Parenteral Nutrition (**PPN**). When done through an IV line going into a larger or central vein, including more chronically, this is called Total Parenteral Nutrition (**TPN**).

Despite all the advances in modern nutritional science, feeding you directly through the blood is just not as good or complete as using your gut. Eating the old fashion way, or even through a feeding tube going straight into the stomach, allows for better nutrition.

Parenteral nutrition is usually considered when we are approaching 5-6 days of inability to feed you using your gut. In the longer term, this therapy is used for individuals who've had bowel surgery, absorption issues, or other reasons where the gut doesn't work. There are specific complications with this type of nutrition, including developing pancreatitis, gallbladder issues, and fungal blood stream infections.

J. Tracheostomy

Tracheostomy is a procedure where an opening is created directly through the neck and into the windpipe (trachea) for you to breathe by way of a short plastic tube inserted into that opening. There are generally two reasons you end up with a tracheostomy. The first reason is that you are on a ventilator too long and aren't able to breathe on your own for the foreseeable future. The second is any one of a set of emergencies such as severe upper airway swelling due to an allergic reaction, a throat tumor, or an emergency airway making traditional intubation through the throat impossible.

Tracheostomies can be done through a fully surgical approach, and also through a puncture and dilation approach. The following describes the second scenario:

After obtaining consent when we talk about bleeding, thyroid damage, loss of airway (asphyxiation), and infection, and you say yes, we determine the difficulty of the procedure and see if it requires an operating room. If it does, your surgeon will schedule a time around their golf game (hope for rain), and takes you to the operating room. Intensivists do not perform this procedure.

If you are skinny and have a long neck, a tracheostomy can be safely done at the bedside in the ICU. Since you are already on a ventilator that is breathing for you, you can be safely sedated.

We perform hand hygiene, don proper attire, clean the area, and drape it with sterile sheets. The operator numbs the area in your neck just underneath the cricoid cartilage ("Adam's apple") and inserts a needle with a negative pressure syringe. Once we get a rush of air back, we pass a guidewire through the needle which goes down your trachea. Another operator is at the head of the bed with a bronchoscope through the endotracheal tube which allows direct visualization of the airway (see section E above for a description of bronchoscopy).

The endotracheal tube is slowly withdrawn while under direct visualization through the bronchoscope until it's just behind the guidewire. The operator at the neck then makes a small incision and passes a set of progressively larger dilators using the guidewire to open a hole in your trachea. After the hole is fully dilated, the more rigid tracheostomy tube is placed through and secured with sutures and a band around your neck. The endotracheal tube is removed and the ventilator tubing is attached directly to the tracheostomy tube – voila!

In an emergency setting, all this is done while you may be undergoing chest compressions, defibrillation, and lots of chaos which carries a high risk of death.

For more chronic applications where you are discharged and otherwise functioning but still unable to use your upper airway, tracheostomies can be converted surgically to permanent openings. This is usually done in the setting of throat cancer surgery, and not in an acute ICU scenario. These types of tracheostomies may include an imbedded valve that allows you to talk while activated, or you may end up using a voice resonator (**electolarynx**) like you see on TV.

> ***ICU Confidential Trach Talk Edition:*** Proceeding to a tracheostomy in the ICU is absolutely a big deal. It usually means you have not been able to recover quickly enough and are now transitioning to a long-term approach with chronic artificial ventilation. Having said this, it is still very possible and, in some ways, safer to wean from life support with a tracheostomy tube. You can be awake and breathing on your own through the tube, as well as speaking through it with the use of a special small valve attached to the tube entrance (a **Passey-Muir Valve** or **PMV**). You can gradually build up strength while you take longer and longer breaks from the ventilator. When you are well enough, the tracheostomy can be replaced for a smaller one, then capped off, and then removed. This typically takes weeks and is done at a **long-term acute care hospital**.

K. Cardioversion / Defibrillation

When the heart beats in an irregular fashion and is causing your blood pressure to drop, we give special medications to try to support you as we figure out and hopefully correct whatever caused this arrhythmia. Sometimes, when your situation is critical, and medications aren't working as quickly as we need them to, we turn to electricity.

Depending on the arrhythmia, triggering the reset button on the heart's electrical system can restore normal rhythm and a life sustaining blood pressure with it. This is done when the ventricles are fibrillating (**ventricular fibrillation** or **v-fib**), or when the top of your heart is just spasming with a very rapid heart rate such as with severe **atrial fibrillation** or **ventricular tachycardia**, or during a **cardiac arrest**.

After obtaining consent where we tell you that basically it's going to hurt and can trigger a terminal arrhythmia, and after you say yes, we place a special conductive pad on the upper right front of the chest and the other on the lower left side of the chest. Sometimes the right pad is placed on your back. It's pretty rare to have actual paddles like you see on television – too much risk to shock ourselves. The pads also do double duty in helping identify the rhythm. Hopefully there's time to give you a little bit of sedation before we press the shock button, because it's going to hurt when we press it.

Depending on the type of arrhythmia, we can use a special shock called **synchronized cardioversion**, such as when we are resetting arrhythmias like atrial fibrillation or unstable ventricular tachycardia, or defibrillation, which delivers a high energy unsynchronized shock. Defibrillation can be done in an emergency, including when you go down at your friendly neighborhood mall or electively where there is time to pre-medicate you and use lower energy levels.

L. Extra-Corporeal Membrane Oxygenation (ECMO)

Extra-Corporeal Mechanical Oxygenation refers to a technology that replaces the function of the lungs (venoveous or **VV-ECMO**) or heart and lungs (veno-arterial or **VA-ECMO**). ECMO is similar to a heart-lung bypass machine in the operating room used during cardiac surgery or heart or lung transplantation. In the ICU, it represents a last-ditch effort to bridge to more definitive therapy best done in young single-organ-problem individuals who were healthy otherwise.

To learn more about ECMO management with some descriptions of how the procedure itself is done, please take a look at Chapter 8: Life Support in the ICU.

M. Targeted Temperature Management/Therapeutic Hypothermia

After sustaining a cardiac arrest, one of the interventions shown to improve neurological function is to decrease your body temperature. After stabilizing the heart through catheterization, cardioversion, or other appropriate intervention, the decision is made to put you under this protocol if your neurological function appears impaired (for example, you are not waking up).

Therapeutic hypothermia, also called targeted temperature management (**TTM**), involves ice packs, cooling blankets, and cold body wraps, and can also involve invasive cooling interventions such as urinary bladder irrigation with cold water. The idea is to prevent fevers and cool the body (and therefore the brain). While there has been debate about how low a temperature we target, this has been consistently shown to improve neurological outcomes and survival after cardiac arrest. Therapeutic hypothermia typically occurs over 48 hours and requires careful monitoring as it can have significant potential complications including electrolyte imbalance, arrhythmia and shock.

N. Blood Transfusions

A number of scenarios may require you to get replacement blood products. These include blood loss, of course, but also may be required when you have an abnormality in how well your blood is clotting (**coagulopathy**). Cancer, chemotherapy, liver disease, and blood thinner overdoses are common scenarios when blood products may be needed.

Depending on the particular deficiency, different blood products are offered. **Packed red blood cells** (**PRBCs**) are the most common replacement when you are bleeding. **Platelets** are a type of circulating cell that helps in coagulation and can also be specifically replaced. If **clotting factor** (chemicals that thicken your blood) deficiencies are in place, **cryoprecipitate** and **fresh frozen plasma** (**FFP**) may be needed.

The blood supply has become incredibly safe from infections. In fact, the most common complication is when you receive the wrong blood type, or when you naturally produce multiple antibodies, making it more difficult to find the right match that your body won't reject. Complications are rare, but may include allergic reactions, fluid overload, and a rapid accumulation of fluid in the lungs called **transfusion related lung injury (TRALI)**.

Transfusing blood products involves multiple checks for compatibility in the blood bank, rigid checks including by two nurses to make sure the right product goes to the right patient, and careful monitoring as these products are being infused.

> ***ICU Confidential Bloody Hell Edition:*** Receiving blood products requires informed consent. If you are a Jehovah's Witness, declining blood may be a religious issue rather than a medical one. We always respect these decisions as part of informed consent, and also recognize that there are some variations on what types of fractions derived from blood may be acceptable (for example, human albumin infusion). We do our best by using interventions to maximize the blood you do have, but even these can sometimes not be enough (otherwise, no one would ever need blood transfusions). As a competent adult, you (or your medical proxy) have the ultimate say in what blood products you receive.

3 Medications in the ICU

While medications are foundational in the interventions you'll get in any part of the hospital, some require very close monitoring and titration that can only be safely done in the ICU. These medications may require minute-to-minute adjustment. Some require a special **central venous catheter** or **arterial catheter**.

The following descriptions are meant to familiarize you with some of the major categories of medications that typically require ICU monitoring. This list is not exhaustive and does not include any of the additional medications you may end up needing which do not need ICU monitoring. Version of these medications can also be used outside the ICU (even chronically at home).

Please keep in mind that depending on where you are in the world, the names of these medications can change, but the functions are similar. Please also keep in mind that this list (like everything in this book) is in no way meant to replace your physician's expert advice.

Please Note: In the lists below, I sometimes include the common trade name(s) alongside the generic names only for recognition, because that's how we refer to them. This is **not** a recommendation for a specific brand.

A. Anti-arrhythmic Medications

Sometimes the heart wants what it wants, and that is to beat to a different drum, or freelance, or go too fast or too slow. When the heart rhythm is abnormal, we call this an **arrhythmia**. When an arrhythmia becomes too slow to keep you conscious (like a **heart block**), or too fast and irregular (like in **atrial fibrillation** with rapid ventricular response or **ventricular tachycardia**), your blood pressure can become dangerously low and must be quickly corrected. Anti-arrhythmic medications exist to do just that. In an urgent situation, they are given intravenously as an IV **bolus** (rapid infusion) or as a continuous IV drip and require careful titration. You usually get an oral medication at the same time or shortly after things are under control with the goal of coming off the IV (so you can leave the ICU). Some examples of anti-arrhythmic medications are as follows:

Adenosine

Used to acutely slow down certain types of rapid heart rates, given as an IV push. Causes a brief pause in the beating of your heart (and ours).

Amiodarone

This is an anti-arrhythmic medication that is a multi-faceted powerhouse, used for dangerous ventricular arrhythmias and difficult to control atrial fibrillation. While it can cause a drop in blood pressure acutely, and has a slew of potential long-term consequences, it is a powerful drug in the ICU. It is usually loaded with an IV bolus followed by a drip followed by a transition to pills.

Cardizem/Diltiazem

IV formulations that can be titrated to control atrial fibrillation when the heart rate is too fast. Oral versions of this medications may be used once stable. This is a calcium channel blocker (nothing to do with osteoporosis).

Esmolol

An IV drip medication that helps control atrial fibrillation with less chance of dangerously dropping your blood pressure. It is a beta-blocker which lowers the effect of adrenaline and helps slow down the heart rate.

Labetolol

IV bolus medication that is used to temporarily control rapid heart rate and very high blood pressure. This is a beta-blocker.

Lidocaine

An oldie but goody used as a backup intravenous agent for certain arrhythmias. It works by blocking sodium channels in the heart which reduces the speed of electrical conduction and controls very fast heart rates caused by certain arrhythmias. It can also be used as a local anesthetic to numb skin and soft tissue.

Magnesium

In cases of low magnesium levels in the blood, replacing this through an IV can correct or prevent a number of dangerous arrhythmias.

Sotalol

Another type of beta-blocker used to treat rapid atrial fibrillation and other arrhythmias.

Cardioversion

This is not a medication, but I'm still including it here since this is a nuclear option in certain arrhythmias where medications aren't working. You undergo an electric shock to the heart to reboot the electrical system (See Appendix II: Common Procedures in the ICU).

> ***ICU Confidential:*** It's important to understand that a rapid heart rate is perfectly normal when your adrenaline levels are high like when you are fighting a critical illness, are very anxious or in pain, or being chased by a bear. We don't try to control this when it's a normal response. Only when the heart rate itself is a problem does it need to be managed. If you see your heart rate is elevated but is in normal (sinus) rhythm as an appropriate response to whatever is going on, it's okay. Also, stop looking at your heart rate on the monitor (it will only stress you out further and lead to an even higher heart rate).

B. Vassopressors/Pressors

When your blood pressure drops too low, your organs don't get enough blood and start to become damaged. This is called being in **shock** or being **hemodynamically unstable.** It can be caused by many things including a heart attack, severe bleeding, an arrhythmia, blood clot in the lung (**pulmonary embolism**) and severe infection (**sepsis**).

As the underlying problem is being worked on, you need an artificial way to get the blood pressure up quickly and in a controlled manner. If you're still in shock after getting enough IV hydration (**fluid resuscitation**) or blood products if you're bleeding, we turn to a handful of IV medications that can raise your blood pressure quickly. Referred to as **pressors**, these medications are essentially forms of adrenaline, flogging your heart to work harder and your blood vessels to constrict so that blood flow is redirected to your essential organs.

The types and dosages of pressors are chosen based on how low the blood pressure is dropping, how much organ damage the low blood pressure is causing, and what is causing the drop in the first place. Low blood pressure from severe infection (**septic shock**) may require a different approach from low blood pressure from heart failure (**cardiogenic shock**).

Pressors have many side effects, including arrhythmias, heart attacks, soft tissue damage, and small blood vessel damage (think ischemia of the fingertips and toes). Unless pressors are used in small doses and only for a short period of time, they need a central venous catheter (see Appendix I: Machines and Things). If you require high dose or multiple pressors, you also benefit from an arterial line so that blood pressure can be monitored directly and continuously. For more information on shock, see Chapter 8: Life Support in the ICU.

Norepinephrine / Levophed® (Levo)

This is the workhorse of the blood pressure support world. It is the Coke® of pressors and usually the first go-to when the blood pressure is dangerously low. Norepi binds to alpha and beta adrenergic ("adrenalin") receptors in the blood vessel walls and the heart, causing the heart to work harder and the blood vessels to constrict thereby increasing the blood pressure. Like all pressors, the higher the dosage the higher the side effects, including life-threatening arrhythmias.

Vasopressin

This is the backup. It constricts (squeezes) the blood vessels to push more blood to the central circulation and therefore to the essential organs. Vassopressin works on increasing intracellular calcium leading to contraction of the muscles in the walls of blood vessels, and also has an anti-diuretic effect. It is sometimes used to decrease the norepinephrine dosing so as to minimize that medication's side effects.

Epinephrine and Phenylephrine

Forms of pure adrenaline, usually given as a third-line additive agent. Sometimes, these medications are used as a small bolus to get you over a short hump (say an acute drop in blood pressure after receiving a sedative or undergoing intubation). These medications combined with the severe shock that requires their use can lead to a high risk of arrhythmias.

Dopamine

This works best if a low heart rate (bradycardia) is part of the problem. It is a precursor to norepinphrine and adrenaline. At higher doses, it works by activating beta-1 adrenergic receptors and constricts blood vessels while raising heart rate It does not work well in raising blood pressure overall. It is not used as a primary pressor.

Midodrine

Although not given as an IV or emergently, this is an oral add-on medication to help get you off IV pressors and to help you tolerate certain procedures like dialysis. It works to constrict blood vessels by activating alpha adrenergic receptors on the smooth muscles in blood vessels. The effect is usually modest.

> ***ICU Confidential 3, 4 and You're Out Edition:*** If you are on 3 or 4 pressors together, it usually means that the underlying infection, heart failure, or whatever else got you to this severity of shock has a smaller and smaller chance of turning around. Things are not going well so make sure you are prepared for anything.

> ***ICU Confidential, Going Low Edition:*** We typically look at blood pressure by combining the upper (**systolic**) and lower (2 times the **diastolic**) blood pressure numbers (and dividing by 3) to calculate the **Mean Arterial Pressure**, or **MAP**. The lower safe cut off is considered ***65 mmHg.*** This number is based on lots of data that suggests that most people need this level of blood pressure to get proper blood supply to their organs.
>
> There are some patients that function just fine at lower blood pressures and have no symptoms. This includes chronic liver disease patients but is also seen in completely healthy patients. If your blood pressure is normally low at home when you are healthy, let us know — it's important that we treat you and not just your number.

C. Fluids

Technically not medications, IV fluids are your first-line treatment and absolutely essential in saving you from shock (especially if it is due to sepsis, trauma or severe dehydration). IV fluids temporarily increase the volume in your blood vessels to keep your blood pressure up and your essential organs perfused. In trauma when you are bleeding out, rapidly initiating blood products and IV fluids makes the difference between life and death. This is also true in severe infection (**sepsis**) as your body undergoes severe inflammation, and the blood pressure drops. Fluids used in resuscitation fall under two main categories:

Crystalloids

A group of intravenous solutions of water, electrolytes, minerals and sometimes sugars used to treat shock and dehydration. Common examples include **Normal Saline (0.9% NaCl), Lactated Ringers®, and Plasma-Lyte®** solutions. Depending on your electrolyte levels, there are a number of variations to meet your needs.

Colloids

These fluids contain large molecules that stay in your blood vessels longer presumably doing a better job in temporarily normalizing your blood pressure. In practice, this is not typically true and colloid solutions are not recommended as first line in most situations. The most common and probably only useful example is IV **albumin**, a protein derived from pooled human blood plasma (from donated blood).

Technically, blood products like concentrated ("packed") red blood cells (PRBCs) are also considered natural colloids and are absolutely essential if you are severely anemic or have low levels of certain blood cells. Blood products are not given as resuscitation fluids if your blood cell levels are normal.

D. Anti-Hypertensives

While low blood pressure can be deadly, high blood pressure can kill you as well. Not just chronic regular high blood pressure, but super high blood pressure, enough to cause organ damage like kidney failure, confusion, stroke, fluid in the lungs (pulmonary edema), and heart failure. Usually occurring in patients that already have high blood pressure at baseline, the regulatory balance is sometimes significantly thrown off. This can happen if you miss your medications, have a high salt diet, miss a dialysis session, or just spontaneously, where the blood pressure acutely rises to the point of giving you severe symptoms.

When high blood pressure (usually > 180/120 mmHg) gives you symptoms like headaches and shortness of breath but not direct organ damage, you have **hypertensive urgency**. When high blood pressure is acutely damaging your organs (brain, heart, kidneys, eyes), you have a **hypertensive emergency,** and this warrants intensive control with IV medications. Some of these medications are also used as anti-arrhythmic medications (see above).

In the ICU, IV anti-hypertensive medications can effectively drop blood pressure in a controlled way. This is important as dropping blood pressure too fast can also be dangerous.

Anti-hypertensives can be used as a continuous titratable IV infusion or as intermittent bolus infusions directly into your blood stream. Oral medications to control blood pressure (pills or tablet versions of the IV drugs) are usually given at the same time, take longer to take effects (hours and days), and are less predictable, but work better to provide long-term control.

Because there are a lot of IV anti-hypertensive medications, I list them here by category.

Vasodilators

Nitroglycerine, nitroprusside, and hydralazine are examples of medications that directly relax or **vasodilate** blood vessels through different mechanisms, thereby lowering systemic blood pressure. They all have their own side effects, and specific medications are preferred depending on the scenario. The biggest complication is if they drop blood pressure too quickly resulting in too large a swing.

Adrenaline Inhibitors / Beta-blockers

Beta-blockers like labetalol and esmolol can be used to decrease blood pressure incrementally by blocking the effects of adrenaline and other stress hormones on the blood vessels and the heart. They have to be monitored carefully as they can slow down the heart rate too much resulting in lowering blood pressure too quickly.

Calcium Channel Blockers

Medications like nicardipine, nimodipine, clevidipine, diltiazem, and verapamil decrease the amount of calcium entering the muscle cells of the heart and blood vessels thereby relaxing them. This decreases blood pressure and heart rate.

ACE Inhibitors

Enalaprilat, a common angiotensin-converting enzyme (ACE) inhibitor, works to decrease blood pressure by decreasing a hormone (angiotensin II) that constricts blood vessels. Examples that can be given orally include captopril, lisinopril, and enalapril. When the blood vessel walls relax, they accommodate more blood volume and drop overall blood pressure.

> ***ICU Confidential, The High Road Edition:*** Just like if you normally live at lower blood pressure, your blood pressure may normally be high. Lots of reasons explain this including genetics, excess weight, and kidney disease. We treat very high blood pressure relative to your baseline blood pressure if you have signs and symptoms of end-organ damage (headaches, worsening kidney function, acute changes in vision, chest pain). We also aim to lower blood pressure in a measured way, meaning that we may not target normal right away.

> ***ICU Confidential, Not Too Low Edition:*** Certain medical conditions like acute stroke can happen because of chronically high blood pressure. An embolic stroke (caused by a blood clot) can also cause the blood pressure to remain high as the body's way of maintaining blood flow to the damaged area. We have different parameters for controlling high blood pressure in this scenario, allowing it to be elevated for a certain period of time.

E. Additional Cardiac Support

If the heart fails, there are chemical ways beyond pressors that can give it a boost. These medications work to improve heart failure in a temporary way as a bridge to something else, such as mechanical support with a left ventricular assist device or heart transplant. Although pressors can make the heart work harder, advanced heart failure medications work primarily on the heart's function, making it work better (improve **contractility**) not just harder. Check out more information in the advanced cardiac support section in Chapter 8: Life Support in the ICU.

Dobutamine (Dobutrex®)

An older but still useful medication to help the heart muscles contract. Complications like low blood pressure and low heart rate limit its use. Dobutamine is available only as an IV infusion, although it can be used continuously through a special pump including at home.

Milrinone (Primacor®)

A more common and effective contractility medication often used as a bridge to heart transplantation, it can sometimes be a destination therapy where people go home with a semi-permanent IV pump.

Dopamine

This medication can be especially useful with low heart rate (**bradycardia**) conditions by helping increase the heart rate. It is a precursor to adrenaline in the heart.

F. Sedation and Pain Control

Sedation is necessary for your comfort and safety. Pain and anxiety control is provided across an array of indications in the ICU. From the discomfort of an endotracheal tube to tolerating procedures and surgical wounds, to controlling severe agitation, a wide array of medications is available.

While pressors, antiarrhythmics, and additional cardiac medications can be managed with the help of a cardiologist, sedation and pain control are primarily controlled by the intensivist. I spend a little more time explaining these here as these more directly affect your quality of life in the ICU. The following sedatives are seen often in the ICU setting:

Dexmedetomidine (Precedex®, or *"dex"*)

This medication is in a class of its own. Initially used during surgery and recovery, dexmedetomidine has become a staple of ICU sedation as a adrenergic receptor agonist (activator). It has limited pain control qualities but works well as a sedative. Dex is rapid onset and offset and can be precisely titrated to get just the right level of sedation. It can be used (very carefully) in non-intubated patients as it does not impact your respiration. Dex is notorious for dropping your heart rate.

Fentanyl

The street drug responsible for so much misery can be useful in the ICU. Its rapid onset and metabolism, and high potency, makes fentanyl valuable during procedures. It's also used as a continuous drip to control the severe pain you may have when recovering from surgery while on a ventilator, typically used together with a sedating medication like propofol or versed. It may be used as a continuous drip, as a bolus, and as a transdermal patch (more for outpatient use).

As a narcotic used in a controlled hospital environment, this medication will make you drowsy and confused, drop your blood pressure, and interfere with your breathing. As an illicit drug abused in the outpatient setting, it will ruin the lives of you and your loved ones and ultimately kill you by overdose.

Haloperidol (Haldol®) and Chlorpromazine (Thorazine®)

These drugs are commonly given in escalating doses for the agitated patient who is in danger of hurting themselves or us when they get severely confused and combative. There remains controversy in how effective they are in reducing harm or improving survival. These antipsychotics calm you down, sometimes even to the point of losing consciousness. They can be given intravenously and intramuscularly. They can cause a drop in blood pressure but don't usually interfere with your ability to breathe. They can cause arrhythmias so an EKG check prior to high dosing is a must.

Ketamine

A sedative, ketamine acts by binding to the NMDA receptor to produce a cataleptic-like state in which you are dissociated from your physical environment. Offering some pain control in lower doses, it can be used as an adjunct to keep you sedated and more comfortable while on the ventilator or during surgical procedures. ICU physicians sometimes refer to this as "vitamin K" or "special K," borrowed from the older street term.

Lidocaine Patch

This version of lidocaine is topically applied for temporary relief of muscle or neuropathic pain. It's a great alternative to narcotics or other systemic drugs and is especially effective for local pain control without altering your sensorium.

Melatonin

Not a strong sedative or hypnotic, melatonin is actually a sleep phase adjuster. The ICU is a great place to ruin your sleep cycle as day turns into night and night into day and sleep comes in erratic spurts. Given about 2 to 3 hours before your expected bedtime, this naturally occurring hormone helps reinforce your regular sleep schedule which helps prevent delirium. It should be combined with doing your best to stick to as normal a sleep schedule as possible in the ICU. More about sleep in Chapter 12: Advice for Getting the Best Experience.

Midazolam (Versed®)/ Alprazolam (Ativan®)

These are benzodiazepines (like Valium® or Xanax®) in IV form commonly used in the ICU for sedation during procedures, as well as in continuous drip form for longer term sedation while on a ventilator. With fast onset but slower to metabolize, these medications are used if anxiety is a larger part of your situation, and if you are expected to be on a ventilator for longer periods.

If you are severely agitated from your anxiety, are at risk for seizures, or if you are withdrawing from alcohol while on a ventilator, this becomes a reasonable choice. Benzodiazepines can be used as a bolus, or as a continuous drip. Alprazolam given in bolus doses, especially for seizures, is another medication in this category.

This class of medications will make you more confused, especially if you are elderly. It can drop your blood pressure, cause respiratory depression, and vomiting. The continuous drip form requires ICU monitoring (and usually being on a ventilator).

Morphine and Hydromorphone (Dilaudid®)

These are similar narcotic drugs used for control of severe pain. In the ICU, they are usually administered intravenously as a bolus, and sometimes as a drip. They can also be used through a **patient-controlled anesthetic (PCA)** pump where you get a basal IV infusion and control bolus dosing using a *happy* button. Each has its special characteristics, including morphine not being used on patients with kidney problems.

Patients who don't respond well to one may respond better to the other. Morphine and hydromorphone are commonly used after surgery, and they both have oral versions that come in short- and long-acting formulations.

Propofol (Diprivan®)

This is an agent now commonly employed for moderate sedation during procedures as well as when putting you on a ventilator with **rapid sequence intubation (RSI)** and for sedation while on a ventilator. Propofol provides sedation quickly to allow full control of your breathing while on a ventilator, and as an adjunct to anesthesia by affecting GABA and NMDA receptors.

Propofol is quickly metabolized and is therefore very useful when we want you to wake up quickly and start breathing on your own, such as after a procedure or surgery. It is also quickly titratable to get more control while you are on life support, and to rapidly minimize this control to safe levels.

Propofol can be given in bolus dosing or as a continuous drip. It is a powerful sedative but does not relieve pain. Never to be used outside a very carefully monitored environment (rest in peace, MJ), this medication will impair your ability to breathe on your own including loss of airway control, can significantly drop your blood pressure, and can also severely raise your triglyceride levels when given in high doses for prolonged periods of time.

> ***ICU Confidential DEA Edition:*** While versions of some of the medications listed above like fentanyl, morphine, hydromorphone, and propofol are explicitly dangerous, they can be indispensable in keeping you safe and comfortable in the ICU during some intensely painful experiences (think surgery, being stabbed with large needles, being intubated). They make what we do to you more tolerable and safer. Our goal is always to minimize their use so that you are not overmedicated - this is a quality marker in the ICU. We titrate them up or down according to your situation, using the lowest dose to get an acceptable effect. If you are on these medications for days or weeks, they will require gradual weaning, but they will not cause addiction.

> ***ICU Confidential Tell Us the Truth Edition:*** When your body is exposed to drugs over a long time it learns how to metabolize them better, effectively making the drug less potent. This is why people with alcohol or drug addiction need higher doses over time to get the same effect. It is very important for you to be honest about any history of prescribed (or illicit) drug use as you may also require higher doses

> of pain and sedative medications in the ICU. It's also very important for us to know this history because withdrawing from narcotics and especially benzodiazepines if they are stopped too quickly can be very difficult and even deadly.

G. Prophylaxis

There are several kinds of medications that help protect you from complications of being laid up and critically ill while in the ICU. It's useful to know some of the main categories of these medications, as receiving them in the ICU is a quality marker.

i. GI Prophylaxis

To protect you against gastric ulcers when you are not eating normally or when you are taking medications that put you at risk, you typically get an acid reducer medication. There are two main types – **histamine blockers (H2B)** and **proton pump inhibitors (PPI)**.

H2 blockers are common anti-acid medications you can get over the counter, including **ranitidine** and **famotidine** (Zantac® and Pepcid®). If your peptic ulcer disease risk is moderately elevated, that's what you get.

If you already had a GI bleed or have other reasons to be higher risk, you get a somewhat stronger version, the PPI, including **pantoprazole** (Protonix®), **omeprazole** (Prilosec®), and the like. Some of these are also now available over the counter. Both H2Bs and PPIs may have side effects and are chosen based on your medical situation.

ii. Deep Vein Thrombosis (DVT) Prophylaxis

You have a higher risk of developing blood clots in the deep (large) veins of your legs when you are not actively moving for a long period of time. These clots can cause swelling, redness, and pain, and can break off and travel to the lungs where they lodge in the pulmonary arteries and prevent blood from reaching the oxygenating part of the lungs. This is called a **pulmonary embolus** and can be very serious, even deadly.

To help prevent this, we give you a mild dose of a blood thinner (**anticoagulant**), usually in the form of an injection under the skin (**subcutaneous**, or **SQ**) in the belly several times a day.

The most common shorter acting medication used for DVT prophylaxis is called **heparin**, and the longer acting version is called **enoxaparin** (Lovenox®). This is pretty standard (another quality marker) and is only withheld if you are regularly walking around (then why are you in the ICU?) or have a high chance of bleeding. Aside from predisposing you to bleeding, blood thinners can have other side effects including decreasing your platelet (blood cell that helps you stop bleeding) count.

You will also get **sequential compression devices (SCDs)** on your legs. These are the strange massage-type stockings connected to an air pump that sequentially squeezes your lower legs to keep the circulation going. Used alone, these don't work nearly as well as when combined with the blood thinners. They do keep you from running away.

iii. Bowel Regimen

While not specific to the ICU, being laid up and fed with liquid tube feeds wreaks havoc on your regular bowel movement schedule and often leads to very uncomfortable constipation. This is why most ICUs will almost automatically put you on stool softeners like **docusate** (Colace®) and/or laxatives like **senna** (Senokot®, ExLax®). Make sure we discontinue these when you inevitably develop diarrhea.

iv. Oral Care

Among the many unpleasant things about being on a ventilator is the inability to maintain good oral hygiene. The plastic tube prevents you from closing your mouth which then gets gummy and gross, and you're not exactly awake to brush your teeth. For these reasons, you may be getting oral care with specially formulated toothpaste as well as **chlorhexidine** (Peridex®), an **antiseptic**.

This can also lower the incidence of ventilator associated pneumonia since the trillions of bacteria now living happily in your mouth are expunged and less likely to travel down your throat and into your lungs. Even if you're not on a ventilator, you may be confused and tired and you don't have access to your normal mouth care, so we do it for you.

v. Skin Breakdown Prophylaxis and Treatment

When immobilized due to critical illness and sedation, it becomes easy to develop pressure sores. These sores, when they commonly affect the buttocks, are called **sacral decubitus ulcers**. They can also affect the heels, any part of the body with bony protrusions under pressure, and any place where equipment like endotracheal tubes and other medical hardware pushes continuously against the skin.

To prevent this, the nurse follows a special turning protocol every two hours designed to prevent continuous pressure on the same part of the skin. Checks for skin breakdown and proper equipment positioning also help prevent this.

Many creams, salves, and dressings exist to prevent worsening and encourage healing of any skin issues. Use of special boots (**podus boots**) that protect the heels, and additional prompt wound care to any place of skin irritation or breakdown, also help. Prevention of pressure sores are a quality marker in the ICU.

Glossary, Jargon, and Slang:

A

Academic (Teaching) Hospital – A hospital where teaching is a priority, staffed by medical students, residents, and sometimes fellows who are working and learning at the same time.

Acute Chest Syndrome – A sickle cell crisis where the abnormally shaped blood cells in *sickle cell disease* block the micro-circulation in the lungs causing low oxygen and lung damage.

Acute Coronary Syndrome (ACS) – A heart attack causing muscle damage that, if severe enough, leads to *heart failure*, low blood pressure, and death.

Acute Respiratory Distress Syndrome (ARDS) – Used to describe respiratory failure due to acute severe inflammation of both lungs; can be caused by severe infection, trauma, or any major injury to the body.

Adenosine – A medication that briefly stops the heart to help identify and sometimes correct certain arrhythmias.

Advanced Cardiovascular Life Support (ACLS) - A protocol initiated during a *Code Blue* that tells the medical team what to do (like *CPR*, emergency drugs, and *intubation*).

Advanced Directives – A set of documents outlining your medical wishes should you become incapacitated, including identifying your *medical proxy*, *code status*, and organ donation wishes.

Advanced Practice Practitioner (APP) - Specially trained medical staff who typically work with a physician but can have significant independence; includes *APRNs*, *CRNAs* and *physician assistants.*

Advanced Practice Registered Nurse (APRN) – An RN who has completed additional education and training that can work independently or with physicians.

Agitated Saline – Sterile *saline* mixed with a small amount of air creating micro-bubbles that act as contrast for *echocardiograms*; not to be confused with angry water.

Airway Box – A (literal) toolbox with equipment needed for intubation, including medications to sedate and paralyze

Airway Protection – Refers to your ability to breathe and swallow normally; when you are in respiratory distress, very confused, in a coma, or are having severe GI bleeding and vomiting, you may lose your ability to protect your airway.

Albumin – A protein normally produced by the liver also available as a formulation given to increase circulating volume; works temporarily and does not treat protein malnutrition as it is quickly metabolized.

Allen Test – Done in preparation for an arterial blood gas puncture to see if your hand has an alternate blood supply in case the target artery gets occluded.

Ambu-bag (Bag Valve Mask or BVM) – A mask meant to fit tightly with an oxygen reservoir bag giving pure oxygen; used in emergency situations to provide mask ventilation in a controlled way prior to intubation.

Amiodarone (Amio) – A common antiarrhythmic medication used in the ICU as well as outside the hospital.

Amyloidosis – A rare condition where amyloid (a type of abnormally folded protein) accumulates in different organs like the heart and brain.

Anaerobic Threshold (AT) – The point at which the body switches from using oxygen for energy to a less "clean" energy source leading to acid over-production; the better your fitness, the higher your AT.

Anaphylaxis – A severe acute allergic reaction that can lead to very low blood pressure (*hemodynamic instability*) and difficulty breathing due to airway swelling.

Anasarca – Total body swelling due to fluid retention in the tissues; may occur from severe heart, kidney, and liver failure, and protein malnutrition.

Anemia – Low level of *red blood cells* or *hemoglobin* decreasing how much oxygen can be transported to tissues.

Angina – A type of chest pain caused by the heart when it is not getting enough blood, such as in an impending heart attack.

Angioedema – Acute swelling of the face and neck usually as part of an allergic reaction; can make it difficult to breathe and lead to asphyxiation if not immediately managed.

Angiography / Angiogram – Dye injected into the arterial system of a particular body-part to check for areas of obstruction or bleeding (*extravasation*).

Angioplasty – Opening clogged arteries like in balloon angioplasty to open coronary arteries.

Anti-arrhythmic Drugs – Medications used to control abnormal heart rhythm (*arrhythmias*).

Antibiotic Sensitivity Panel – A lab test done on bacterial cultures identifying which antibiotics would work best.

Anticoagulation – Giving blood thinners to prevent blood clots while critically ill, or to treat blood clots that have already formed.

Antiseptic – A chemical used to sterilize the skin surface or operating field.

Aorta – The large artery coming from the left *ventricle* of the heart supplying the body with oxygen-rich blood.

Aortic Valve – One-way heart valve between the left *ventricle* and the *aorta*.

Arrhythmia – Any irregularity in the rhythm of the heart.

Arterial Blood Gas (ABG) – A sample of arterial blood used to directly measure oxygen, carbon dioxide, and acid (pH) levels; can also report some electrolyte and hemoglobin levels.

Arterial Line (A-line) – A catheter that goes into an artery allowing for direct and continuous measurement of blood pressure, as well as giving access to collect *arterial blood gases*.

Arteriovenous (AV) Fistula – Abnormal connection between a larger artery and vein; may be surgically created for dialysis.

Arteritis – Inflammation of the arteries typically caused by the immune system.

Artery – Any blood vessels going away from the heart; are muscular and able to constrict for localized blood pressure control.

Artificial (Mechanical) Ventilation – The process of having a machine (*ventilator*) breathe for you; considered the main type of life support.

Ascites – Fluid buildup in the abdominal cavity typically caused by liver failure, cancer, heart conditions or infection.

Atrial Fibrillation (Afib, AF) – A common *arrhythmia* that can cause your heart rate to be very fast and irregular; may require medications or *cardioversion* to slow and convert it back to normal.

Atrial Flutter – Similar to *Afib*, an arrhythmia where the atria are beating in an abnormal way that can lead to very fast heart rates.

Atrium (cardiac) – The top chambers of the heart, right and left.

Attending – Senior physician ultimately in charge of your care.

Auto-Immune – Caused by your own immune system.

Autonomy – The principle that patients should be able to make up their own minds about medical interventions after being fully informed and without coercion.

Autopsy – A protocolized examination of a dead body; usually an extensive evaluation of the body and internal organs although it may be limited to external examination depending on the circumstances.

B

Bacteria – Microbes that can attack the body and cause infections.

Bag Valve Mask (Ambu-Bag) – A mask meant to fit tightly with an oxygen reservoir bag giving pure oxygen; used in emergency situations to provide mask ventilation in a controlled way prior to intubation.

Baker Act (Involuntary Hold) – Allows the medical team to keep you from leaving the hospital (for up to 72 hours) if you are a danger to yourself or others, mainly in the context of psychiatric conditions.

Basic Life Support (BLS) – A protocol used to identify someone acutely struggling, get help, initiate CPR, and apply a defibrillator.

Basic Metabolic Panel (BMP) – A common blood test showing electrolyte levels and kidney function.

Best Case/Worst Case – An approach to helping you decide on a procedure or code status based on the best and worst-case scenarios and the probability of each.

Beta-Blockers – A class of medications used to slow down the heart rate and decrease blood pressure.

Bi-level Positive Airway Pressure (BPAP) - Airflow delivered through a tight-fitting mask with a high pressure as you breathe in (inspiratory or IPAP) and a low pressure as you breathe out (expiratory or EPAP); may be temporarily used as an external ventilator or for chronic conditions like *obstructive sleep apnea* and *obesity hypoventilation syndrome*.

Bilirubin – A yellow waste product from normal breakdown of red blood cells; processed by the liver.

Blood Gas – A shorter term for *Arterial Blood Gas* (*ABG*) to, you know, save you time when you say it.

Blood Pressure (BP) – How much force or pressure is in your blood vessels.

Blood Urea Nitrogen (BUN) - A measure of kidney function, the higher the worse.

Bougie – A thin, flexible plastic rod used to assist in difficult *intubations*.

Bowel Ischemia – Not enough blood flow to keep bowel tissue healthy; can lead to bowel death and perforation. This can occur due to a blood clot occluding the arterial blood supply, and/or very low blood pressure in the setting of vascular disease.

Bowel Regimen – A set of interventions used to prevent constipation, a common complication of being critically ill; usually consists of a stool softener, laxative and sometimes fiber.

Bradycardia – An *arrhythmia* where the heart rate is too slow.

Brain Attack - Used to describe a *stroke* or *cerebrovascular accident*.

Brain Death – Irreversible loss of all brain function, including the brain stem; death (except in NJ).

Broad Spectrum Antibiotics – Wide ranging antibiotics designed to kill many different bacteria used when we don't know the exact type of the bacteria causing infection.

Bronchitis – Inflammation of the airways (bronchi) in the lungs typically from infection; may progress to pneumonia.

Bronchoalveolar Lavage – A *bronchoscopy* procedure where sterile saline is flushed inside a part of the lung and suctioned back for analysis.

Bronchoscopy (bronch) – A procedure involving a thin flexible tube with a fiberoptic camera inserted through the back of the throat, past the vocal cords, and into the main airways; may be used to take biopsies, clean out mucus, and mine for an aspirated peanut (or bitcoin).

Bronchus / Bronchi (pl) – Tube(s) in the lungs stemming from the windpipe delivering air to and from the functional lung units.

Bureau of Vital Statistics – Government agency responsible for keeping death records including death certificates; also keeps birth and marriage certificates (they do it all!).

C

Cancer – Cells that become abnormal and grow out of control.

Capillaries – Microscopic blood vessels connecting the arteries and the veins.

Cardiac Arrest – A medical emergency where the heart stops beating or stops beating effectively.

Cardiac Care Unit (CCU) - A specialized ICU caring for patients with heart problems.

Cardiac Catheterization – A procedure used to evaluate the coronary arteries for blockages, open them (*angioplasty*), and place a *cardiac stent*; uses a catheter passed through the arteries while injecting contrast and taking X-rays.

Cardiac Stent – A tiny mesh-like tube permanently placed in a coronary artery at the site of a blockage to keep it open.

Cardiogenic Shock – Dangerously low blood pressure due to *heart failure*.

Cardiomyopathy – Abnormality of the heart muscle; may be due to *coronary artery disease* (*ischemic*) or to very large size (*hypertrophic*).

Cardiopulmonary Criteria for Death – The permanent cessation of heart and lung function.

Cardiopulmonary Resuscitation (CPR) – Rhythmically compressing the chest and providing other measures to save you when your pulse is gone. This is traumatic if done correctly, broken ribs and all. Part of *BLS/ACLS*.

Cardiorenal Syndrome – When heart failure causes kidney failure, and vice-versa.

Cardioversion – A procedure where electric shock is delivered to the heart to convert it from an abnormal rhythm like *ventricular fibrillation* (*defibrillation*) or *atrial fibrillation* (*synchronized cardioversion*).

Cardizem – A common antiarrhythmic drug used to slow down an overly rapid heart rate.

Case Manager – Assists in communication, insurance questions, and arrangements for care after the ICU.

Centers for Medicare and Medicaid Services (CMS) – Federal agency responsible for administering the Medicare and Medicaid programs.

Central Line / Central Venous Catheter – A large *intravenous* catheter that is placed in a main or central (large) *vein*.

Cerebrospinal Fluid (CSF) – Fluid surrounding your spine and inside the *ventricles* in the brain.

Cerebrovascular Accident (CVA) – A stroke caused by a blood clot (*embolic*) or bleed (*hemorrhagic*) causing localized damage to the brain; the subsequent increased pressure and swelling from inflammation can cause global damage to the brain.

Charge Nurse – The nursing team leader for the shift; first go-to in addressing concerns with your nurse.

Chest Tube – A catheter going through the chest wall to evacuate fluid, puss, blood, or air from inside the chest cavity; may be a small *pig-tail* catheter or a larger, more rigid surgically-placed plastic tube.

Chlorhexidine – An antiseptic used to sterilize the skin for procedures; also used as part of a mouthwash to provide oral care, including while intubated.

Cholangitis – Inflammation of the bile ducts in the liver; may be caused by infection, gallstones, or autoimmune conditions.

Choppa – An aircraft that uses top-mounted rotating blades to fly away from danger; as in, "*get to the choppa.*"

Chronic Obstructive Pulmonary Disease (COPD) – A chronic progressive inflammatory lung disease causing breathing difficulties.

Cirrhosis – Scarring of the liver from alcohol, fatty deposits, viruses, or auto-immune causes, eventually leading to liver failure.

Circulatory System – Consisting of the heart (pump) and the blood vessels (plumbing), the system that circulates blood throughout the body.

Closed ICU – An ICU where the intensivist physician has the ultimate responsibility for your care; all orders and recommendations go through the intensivist.

Clostridioides difficile (C. Dif) – An infection of the gastrointestinal tract that can cause severe diarrhea and gut inflammation; highly contagious requiring hand washing (not chemical hand cleaners). Risk increases with the use of certain antibiotics.

Clotting Factors – An array of chemicals mostly made in the liver needed to *coagulate* (thicken) your blood; different medications and disorders can deplete your clotting factors. May be replaced with blood product transfusions.

Coagulation – Your ability to clot blood so as not to bleed all over us.

Coagulopathy – A problem with blood clotting predisposing you to bleed.

Code Status – A medical directive which informs us of your wishes for attempt at resuscitation should you die; see DNR, DNI, Full, CMO.

Code (Blue) – You are dying or have died, initiating a resuscitation protocol where we perform chest compressions, deliver electric shock to the heart, intubate, and so forth.

Colonoscopy – A procedure where a flexible scope is inserted through the anus and up the rectum, sigmoid, and large intestine; may be used to identify sources of bleeding, inflammation, obstruction, and doge coin.

Colostomy – A surgical procedure where the colon is diverted through the abdominal wall allowing stool to come out of the colon into a *colostomy bag.* Called a *diverting* colostomy when used for wound control.

Colostomy Bag – The bag attached over a colostomy to collect the stool.

Coma – A deep state of unconsciousness with an inability to arouse, caused by a stroke, severe lack of oxygen or low blood pressure, or other severe medical condition; may be medically induced such as for surgery or to keep you breathing with the ventilator.

Comfort Measures Only (CMO) – A designation in your care where all treatments are exclusively meant to provide comfort; what happens in *hospice.*

Complete Blood Count (CBC) – A common blood test that measures the types and numbers of cells in your blood.

Comprehensive Metabolic Panel (CMP) – A common blood test showing electrolyte levels, as well as kidney and liver function levels.

Computer Tomography (CT) – An imaging test involving multiple X-rays collected through a special machine that allows for detailed images of most parts of the body; may be combined with IV contrast to look for blood clots, bleeding, and many other abnormalities.

Condition – A somewhat subjective summary of your medical situation condensed to one word: Good, Fair, Guarded, Critical, Expired (like milk but worse).

Congestive Heart Failure (CHF) – When the heart is unable to pump efficiently leading to fluid buildup in the soft tissues causing leg swelling (*edema*), and in the lungs causing shortness of breath.

Consultant – A specialist like a cardiologist or pulmonologist giving advice to the primary medical team.

Continuous Positive Airway Pressure (CPAP) – Pressurized airflow provided through a mask to keep the back of the throat open while you sleep; treats a condition called *obstructive sleep apnea* (*OSA*).

Continuous Veno-venous Hemodialysis (CVVHD) – A slow form of blood *dialysis* performed continuously (instead of only 3-4 hours per session); decreases the risk of low blood pressure but requires ICU monitoring.

Contractility – How well the heart is squeezing to pump blood.

Contusion – Bruise.

Coronary Arteries – The blood vessels supplying the heart with freshly oxygenated blood.

Coronary Artery Bypass Graft (CABG) – Open heart surgery that grafts healthy blood vessels to replace blocked coronary arteries.

Corpak® – A type of feeding tube.

Costophrenic – The area in the lower part of your back towards your sides where the bottom of the rib cage is; tenderness in this area may signify a kidney infection. Fluid in the *costophrenic angle* as seen on an X-ray may signify fluid in the chest cavity below the lungs.

Craniotomy (Crani) – An operation involving opening the skull.

Crash Cart – A cart on wheels that has all the drugs and typical supplies used in attempting resuscitation or providing *ACLS* in a *Code Blue* situation.

Creatinine – A measure of kidney function, the higher the worse.

Cricothyroidotomy (Crike) – A surgical procedure used to establish an airway directly through your neck when conventional intubation attempts fail; a last-ditch emergency procedure.

Critical Care – Intensive care.

Critical Care Registered Nurse (CCRN) – Specially trained critical care nurse with a certification based on training and expertise.

D

Death – Defined as irreversible loss of all brain function (*brain death*) and of the heart and lungs (*cardiopulmonary death*).

Death Certificate – A very important legal document noting when and from what you died.

Debride – Removing dead or damaged tissue from a wound.

Decerebrate Posturing – A reflex characterized by stiff back, straight arms with flexed wrists, clenched fists and straight legs, typically indicating severe damage to the brain stem.

Declaration of Death – A protocol to confirm death including checking for lack of a pulse, breathing, and responsiveness; verifies the time and place of death.

Deconditioned – Losing strength and muscle mass from being chronically sick and laid up in bed.

Decorticate Posturing – A reflex characterized by stiff back, arms bent towards the chest, clenched fists and straight legs, typically indicating severe brain damage.

Deep Tendon Reflexes – Involuntary muscle contractions triggered by tendon trauma, like the leg kicking when you tap just below the knee; may be present in brain death as it involves only the spinal cord.

Deep Vein Thrombosis (DVT) - A blood clot in a larger vein typically in the legs causing pain, redness, and swelling; can dislodge and travel to the lungs causing a *pulmonary embolus.*

De-escalation of Care – In the ICU, withdrawal of technological support including the *ventilator, dialysis* and any other artificial means of *life-support*; occurs when converting to *Comfort Measures Only* or *hospice.*

Defibrillation – Applying an electric shock to the heart to reset and correct an *arrhythmia.*

Defibrillator – A medical device used for *defibrillation.*

Delirium – Waxing and waning confusion usually caused by medications, lack of sleep, and just being very sick in the ICU; scarry to experience, temporary in nature.

Dementia – A progressive and terminal neurological condition causing memory loss and impacting cognitive skills; examples include Alzheimer's, vascular dementia, Lewy body dementia, and frontotemporal dementia.

Destination Therapy – A final treatment option to improve and sustain life.

Dexmedetomidine (Dex) – A potent IV sedative that affects breathing less; can cause a slow heart rate.

Diagnosis Related Group (DRG) – A system that groups patients with similar diagnoses and complexities together to determine a common payment for services.

Dialysis – A procedure that replaces kidney function by exchanging blood (*hemodialysis*) or putting in special fluid and then taking it out of your abdomen overnight (*peritoneal dialysis*); can be used to remove excess fluid, adjust electrolytes, and remove certain toxins.

Diastole – The part of the cardiac cycle where the heart muscles relax allowing the heart chambers to refill with blood.

Diastolic Blood Pressure – The amount of force, measured in mmHg (millimeters of mercury), in your circulatory system during heart relaxation; the bottom number of your blood pressure.

Dietician – A specialist in assessing your nutritional needs and how to deliver them; requires additional training and credentials beyond *nutritionist.*

Direct Admission – Being admitted to the hospital directly from another hospital or even from home, bypassing the ER; can be more convenient but also worse because the ER has a very important role in your evaluation.

Disimpaction – The process of manually removing hard stool from the rectum.

Diuretic – A medication that makes you urinate more; used to treat *fluid overload* in *congestive heart failure.*

Dobhoff® Tube – A feeding tube that goes through the nose to the stomach.

Dobutamine – A potent IV medication that enhances heart function but can also drop blood pressure.

Do Not *Attempt* Resuscitation (DNR) – A designation where attempts at ACLS (like chest compressions, defibrillation, or intubation) are not initiated if you are dying/dead.

Do Not Intubate (DNI) – A designation where you would not want to be put on a ventilator.

Dopamine – A potent medication that increases blood pressure and heart rate.

Docusate – A common stool softener given as part of the bowel regimen to prevent constipation while critically ill; common trade name is Colace®.

Double Effect / Intent – An ethical principle allowing an action to be morally permissible even if it has a secondary bad effect, as long as the bad effect was not intended; may be applied to causing pain during a lifesaving procedure or giving medication to relieve severe pain in a terminal condition even if it hastens death.

Double-Lumen Endotracheal Tube – A special type of breathing tube with two ends; may be used to selectively ventilate the left or right lung.

Downgrade – Patients who are stable enough to leave the ICU are downgraded to a lower level of care like the *Intermediate Care Unit* (*IMCU*) or *telemetry*; a good thing as this means you are getting better.

E

Echocardiogram (Echo) – An ultrasound of your heart showing general muscle size and function, heart valves, and estimated pressures; may be on the chest surface (transthoracic echo or TTE) or through the esophagus (transesophageal or TEE).

ECPR (ECMO CPR) – Applying extracorporeal membrane oxygenation during a code blue.

Edema – Swelling, such as in the legs (soft tissue edema) or the lungs (*pulmonary edema*).

Electrocardiogram (ECG or EKG) – A rapid test that looks at the electrical activity of the heart using small electrodes placed on the skin.

Electroencephalogram (EEG) – Used to assess electrical activity at the surface of the brain using an array of electrodes stuck to your scalp; used to diagnosed seizure, sleep staging, brain death, and more.

Electrolarynx – A voice modulator held up to the neck to allow patients who have a tracheostomy to talk.

Electronic Intensive Care Unit (eICU) – A remotely monitored ICU where the intensivist is at a telemedicine center looking at you with a camera and seeing your vital signs electronically.

Embolism – Refers to a blockage typically caused by a clot as in *embolic stroke* or *pulmonary embolism;* rarely can consist of air in a blood vessel (air embolism).

Emergency Medical Treatment and Labor Act (EMTALA) – A federal law requiring Medicare-participating hospitals to provide a medical screening exam (MSE) and stabilizing treatment to anyone needing emergency care, regardless of ability to pay or insurance status.

Emergency Room / Department (ER/ED) – A dedicated part of the hospital where acutely ill patients come for care; free-standing ERs also exist from which you are transferred to an affiliated hospital by ambulance if you require admission.

Empyema – Pus in the chest cavity indicating severe infection.

Encephalopathy – Brain dysfunction leading to confusion and even coma; can be caused by infection, toxins, strokes, and just being generally sick (toxic).

Endobronchial Blocker – A special tool used in bronchoscopy to block off an airway; typically used to contain bleeding.

Endocarditis – Inflammation of the heart's inner lining (endocardium) and heart valves, typically from infection.

Endoscopy - A procedure where a scope is inserted through the back of the throat and into the esophagus and then the stomach; may be used to identify sources of bleeding, take biopsies, and mine for etherium.

Endotracheal Tube (ETT) – A plastic tube placed through your mouth (rarely through the nose) down your throat, and through the vocal cords to the *trachea* (windpipe) so a ventilator can be attached to breathe for you; an artificial airway.

Enoxaparin – A longer acting blood thinner given under the skin to prevent or treat blood clots; the common trade name is Lovenox®.

Enteral Nutrition – Food the old-fashioned way, using your own gut; as opposed to *parenteral nutrition* where nutrition is provided directly into the blood stream.

Epiglottis – A small, leaf-shaped, cartilaginous flap located in the throat behind the tongue and in front of the larynx; acts as a valve, closing off the airway (*trachea*) during swallowing to prevent food and liquid from entering the lungs.

Epiglottitis – Inflammation of the *epiglottis* which may cause airway closure, causing severe sore throat, painful swallowing, and difficulty breathing.

Epinephrine (Epi) – A potent medication that acutely increases blood pressure and constricts blood vessels.

Escalation of Care – Increasing the amount or degree of medical support.

Esophageal Varices – Abnormally enlarged, swollen veins in the lower *esophagus,* usually occurring in individuals with severe liver disease (*cirrhosis*); may burst and cause severe bleeding.

Esophagus – The part of the gastrointestinal tract that connects the throat to the stomach; involved in swallowing.

Ethics – An accepted set of rules for behavior and morals governing society.

Euthanasia – *Physician assisted suicide* where medications are prescribed to end a patient's life in the context of an end stage terminal illness; legal in some States with many safeguards. Also, young people in Asia.

Euvolemic – Having a well-balanced amount of fluid in the body.

Extracorporeal Membrane Oxygenation (ECMO) – The process of taking blood out of your body, adding oxygen and removing carbon dioxide, and then returning it to your body. *Venovenous (VV) ECMO* replaces the function of the lungs; *Venoarterial (VA) ECMO* replaces the functions of the lungs and the heart.

Extravasation – IV medication leaking into the soft tissue when the vein breaks; may cause severe damage if medication is caustic.

Extubation – The process of removing the breathing (*endotracheal*) tube and discontinuing the *ventilator.*

F

Factors – Refers to chemicals produced by the liver to help with blood clotting (*coagulation*); may be replaced by donated blood products.

Failure to Thrive – Withering away little by little; a slow-motion dying process.

Fellow – A physician in sub-specialty training; for critical care training, they would have already completed full training in Internal Medicine or Anesthesia.

Fiberoptic Endoscopic Evaluation of Swallowing (FEES) – A procedure to evaluate swallowing using a fiberoptic cable to directly visualize the vocal cords while you swallow foods of different consistencies.

Fibrosis – Accumulation of fibrous connective tissue in organs causing scarring, as in fibrosis of the lungs or liver.

Fluid Overload – Having too much fluid in your body causing fluid build-up (*edema*) in your soft tissues and lungs.

Fluid Resuscitation – Where we give you lots of *IV fluids* to respond to low blood pressure, such as in *septic shock.*

Fluids – Referring to intravenous formulations of *IV* liquid containing different combinations of salt, electrolytes, and sugars used to increase your blood volume and to mix with medications; examples include Normal Saline (NS), Half-normal Saline, 5% Dextrose, Lactated Ringers (LR), Plasma-Lyte®, and others.

Fluoroscopy (Fluoro) – An X-ray technique where multiple X-rays are taken in rapid sequence to create a movie of sorts; used in certain procedures like *cardiac catheterizations* and *angiograms* as well as to check your swallowing.

Foley Catheter – A soft tube going through your *urethra* (opening where urine comes out) and into the urinary bladder; has an inflatable reservoir at the end to keep it in place that can cause a lot of damage if you try to pull it out without first collapsing the reservoir.

Full Code – A designation where if you die, we perform *ACLS* (*CPR*, *defibrillations*, IV medications, *ventilator*) to try and *resuscitate* you.

Functional Status – A general assessment of how you perform day to day functions such as dressing, eating, walking, etc.; correlates with survival in medical diseases like cancer, heart failure, organ transplant and more.

Fungemia – Fungus in the blood stream; usually a very serious type of infection requiring prolonged anti-fungal medications.

G

Gamma Camera – A nuclear medicine imaging device used for essential tests like *V/Q* and *PET* scans.

Gastroenteritis – Inflammation of the gastro-intestinal track, typically caused by infection.

Generic Name – The name of a drug given by the company creator that can then be used by other manufacturers once the patent has expired.

Glioma – The most common type of brain tumor.

Goal Directed Medical Therapy (GDMT) - A set of cardiac medications used to treat *heart failure with reduced ejection fraction* (*HFrEF*).

Goals of Care (GOC) – Refers to things like code status and end of life care.

Good Samaritan – A bystander that performs lifesaving interventions in an emergency; is generally protected from liability (as in *Good Samaritan Laws*).

Gram-Negative Bacteria – A group of bacteria that includes E. Coli and Pseudomonas.

Gram-Positive Bacteria – A group of bacteria that includes staph and strep.

Gram-Stain – Refers to initial information on the type of bacteria present in a blood or other body sample; tells us the general category of bacteria such as *gram-negative* or *gram-positive* to help guide antibiotics.

H

Hand Hygiene – Washing or applying chemical cleaner to hands.

Health Care Proxy/Surrogate – The person(s) you assign to make medical decisions on your behalf if you are unable to do so.

Health Insurance Portability and Accountability Act (HIPAA) – A federal law synonymous with protecting your confidentiality and defining how your health information is shared.

Heart Failure (HF) – Used to describe the failing heart, categorized as HF with preserved (*HFpEF*) or reduced ejection fraction (*HFrEF*), each treated somewhat differently.

Heel Ulcers – Pressure sores on the heel of the foot.

Hematocrit (Hct) – The percentage of total blood volume composed of red blood cells; used to gauge *anemia*.

Hematoma – Abnormal collection of blood in tissue or organ.

Hemodialysis (HD) – The process of taking blood out of the body, filtering it, removing excess fluid from it, and returning it to the body.

Hemodynamically Stable/Unstable – Refers to how controlled your blood pressure and heart rate are.

Hemodynamics – Refers to the blood pressure and heart rate, the factors that support your circulation.

Hemoglobin (Hgb) – An iron-rich protein in red blood cells that transports oxygen; used to gauge *anemia*.

Hemorrhage – Bleeding.

Hemorrhagic Shock – Dangerously low blood pressure due to bleeding.

Heparin – A common blood thinner used to prevent blood clots (given under the skin several times a day) or to treat blood clots, heart attacks, and some strokes (given as an IV infusion); extracted from pig intestines, really!

Hepatitis – Inflammation of the liver; may be from viral infection, auto-immune, or other causes.

Hepatobiliary Iminodiacetic Acid (HIDA) Scan – A nuclear medicine test that helps evaluate the liver, gallbladder, and bile ducts; requires injection of a very small amount of radiotracer.

Hepatopulmonary Syndrome – When liver failure takes down your lungs.

Hepatorenal Syndrome – When liver failure takes down your kidneys.

High Flow Oxygen – Extra oxygen delivered at a high rate through a special cannula; has one setting for percent oxygen, and another for rate of gas flow in liters per minute.

Hospice – Technically a health benefit, this is a type of care that focuses on quality of life and comfort in patients who are terminally ill; appropriate when the underlying medical condition is no longer treatable, or the treatments are unacceptable to the patient, and the expected life span is 6 months or less.

Hospital-Based Outpatient Clinic (HBOC) – A clinic operated directly by a hospital following stricter guidelines; a way to charge your insurance higher rates for your outpatient visit.

Hospitalist – Internal medicine physician who cares for hospitalized patients; the main physician taking care of you in the hospital wards.

House Staff – Physicians in training, including *interns*, *residents*, and *fellows*, who do most of the doctor's work (while they learn), taking care of you in the hospital.

Hypercarbia – High blood carbon dioxide levels.

Hypertension – High blood pressure.

Hypertensive Urgency/Emergency – Very high blood pressure causing symptoms/organ damage.

Hyperthermia – High body temperature.

Hypertrophic – Enlarged or overgrown, as in hypertrophic *cardiomyopathy* (abnormal enlargement of the heart).

Hypotension – Low blood pressure.

Hypothermia – Low body temperature.

Hypothyroidism – Low thyroid levels.

Hypovolemic – Not enough fluid in the body, such as in the setting of severe dehydration or bleeding.

Hypoxia – Low oxygen levels in tissues and organs.

I

ICU Bundle – A protocolized group of interventions shown to improve your ICU outcome; includes elements like daily *sedation vacations*, *ventilator weaning* trials, scheduled pain management, and *delirium* assessment.

Ileus – A functional (non-mechanical) obstruction of the bowel.

Impella® – An advanced heart support device placed through the artery across the *aortic valve* that continuously pumps blood providing an extra push of blood flow to assist the failing heart; comes in different "strengths" and is considered higher support than an *intra-aortic balloon pump (IABP)*.

Informed Consent – The concept that patients must be informed about the risks and benefits of a procedure and must give consent before having the procedure; may not apply in an emergency.

Inpatient – Hospitalized patient.

Intensive Care Unit (ICU) – A specially equipped hospital ward where critically ill patients are cared for with close monitoring, specialized care, and advanced expertise.

Intensivist – A physician with specialized training and experience in taking care of ICU patients.

Intermediate Care Unit (IMCU) – A level of care just below the ICU where you have cardiac and other monitoring and a smaller nurse to patient ratio than other areas of the hospital, but not to the level of the ICU.

Intern – A physician in their first year of practical training after completing medical school; a junior member of the *house staff*.

Interventional – Subspecialist with additional training in procedure skills; examples include interventional radiologist, cardiologist, and pulmonologist.

Intra-Aortic Balloon Pump (IABP) – An advanced cardiac support device that is placed through the artery into the aorta; inflates when the heart relaxes and provides an extra push of blood flow to assist the failing heart.

Intra-arterial Line (A-line) – A catheter that goes into an artery allowing for direct and continuous measurement of blood pressure, as well as giving access to arterial blood gas samples.

Intracranial Pressure (ICP) Monitor – A pressure sensor placed through a small opening in the skull to monitor the pressure in the skull.

Intraosseous (IO) Catheter – A catheter that is drilled directly into the bone marrow when an *IV* is difficult to get.

Intravenous (IV) – A catheter that goes into a vein to deliver medications and fluids.

Intravenous Contrast – Dye injected into blood vessels for various imaging tests; may contain iodine.

Intubation – The process of placing an endotracheal tube into your windpipe (*trachea*) to connect you to the *ventilator*.

Involuntary Hold (Baker Act) – Allows the medical team to keep you from leaving the hospital (for up to 72 hours) if you are a danger to yourself or others, mainly in the context of psychiatric conditions.

Ischemia – Not getting enough blood supply to tissue or organ.

J

Jaundice – A yellowing of the skin and eyes as a result of the liver failing to break down *bilirubin*, a yellow product of red blood cell breakdown; may be a sign of liver dysfunction.

K

Ketamine – A powerful sedative used in the ICU to control pain including while being on a ventilator.

Koala – An adorable Australian marsupial; a word used as filler to take up space in an index.

L

Labetalol – A common heart medication used to control high blood pressure and heart rate.

Lactate – A blood test indicating level of tissue inflammation due to not enough blood supply, as in *septic shock*.

Laryngeal Mask Airway (LMA) – A way to temporarily secure the airway and provide ventilation when endotracheal *intubation* is too difficult or only a short time on the ventilator is expected (such as during a procedure).

Laryngoscope – A device used to perform *laryngoscopy*, often with a camera transmitting video to the operator.

Laryngoscopy – A procedure used to examine the back of your throat down to your vocal cord with a special device that may also have a camera; used to assist with *intubation*.

Left Heart Catheterization (LHC) – Using catheter directed dye injections to visualize the left side of the heart as well as the *coronary arteries*.

Left Ventricular Device (LVAD) – A mechanical advanced heart therapy device that augments the push of the heart's left *ventricle*.

Length of Stay (LOS) – The duration of your stay in the ICU or hospital; the shorter the better (unless it's because you died).

Leukemia – Blood cancer of which there are several types.

Levophed® (Levo) – Trade name for norepinephrine, a potent *pressor* medication used to raise dangerously low blood pressure.

Liberated (ICU) – Extubated and disconnected from the ventilator.

Licensed Clinical Social Worker (LCSW) – A mental health professional with a master's degree in social work, specializing in clinical practice.

Lidocaine – A common antiarrhythmic in the ICU; also used as a topical numbing agent.

Line – Refers to an *intravenous* (*IV*) catheter; typically, a large (*central*) catheter that goes into a major blood vessel or artery

Line Infection – Infection from an IV catheter.

Locked In Syndrome – Rare neurologic disorder causing total muscle paralysis while sparing consciousness; spares vertical eye movement or blinking. Also, overconfidence in teenagers or young adults.

Long-Term Acute Care Hospital (LTACH) – A hospital environment equipped to provide long-term (30 day) hospital care, usually after the acute phase of recovery in a regular hospital; common scenarios include need for long-term antibiotics, wound management, ventilator weaning, and complex rehabilitation services.

Lumbar Puncture (LP) – A procedure where a needle is inserted between the vertebrae in your lower back to get a sample of *cerebrospinal fluid*.

Lymphatic System – A system of circulation that is part of the immune system that collects fluid and metabolic byproducts outside the blood circulation.

Lymph Node – Part of the lymphatic system, these are centralized nodules that collect cellular and immune by-products; may get enlarged during infections, cancer, and other inflammatory states.

Lymphoma – Cancer of the lymphatic system; may be chronic and smoldering or acute and immediately dangerous.

M

Magnetic Resonance Cholangiopancreatography (MRCP) – A special *MRI* using dye to visualize the bile and pancreatic ducts.

Magnetic Resonance Imaging / Angiography (MRI/MRA) – A special radiology test using magnetic fields that allows for excellent pictures of solid organs and bones; may be combined with special contrast to allow for blood vessel visualization.

Mean Arterial Pressure (MAP) – The average of your *systolic* (top number) plus 2 times the *diastolic* (bottom number) blood pressure divided by 3; felt to better represent blood perfusion of your organs. For a bp of 120/80 it would be (120 + 80x2)/3 = 87; the low cutoff is generally considered 65 mmHg.

Medical Examiner – A specialized physician, usually a *pathologist*, who investigates suspicious deaths to determine the cause and manner.

Medical Intensive Care Unit (MICU) – Where critically ill medical patients are taken care of; other types of critically ill patients can be cared for in the specialized ICU specific to their issues (like surgical or trauma ICUs).

Metastatic Disease – When cancer spreads beyond its initial location, it is considered metastasized and in a more advanced stage.

Midazolam – A potent IV sedative; type of benzodiazepine.

Mid-flow Oxygen – A middle range of oxygen support.

Mid-line – An intravenous catheter placed in a larger vein (but not as large as a *central line*) using ultrasound as a guide; also, the center line anatomically.

Midodrine – An oral medication that mildly increases blood pressure; often used in dialysis patients.

Milrinone – A potent IV infused medication that enhances heart function.

Mitral Heart Valve – One-way valve between the left *atrium* and left *ventricle*.

Mixed Venous Oxygen Saturation (SvO2) – The percentage of oxygen in the blood returning to the right side of the heart, optimally obtained from a *pulmonary artery catheter* and used to estimate the overall heart function (higher is better).

Modifiable Risk Factors – Things about your health you can change, like weight, fitness level, type of diet. Age is not a modifiable risk factor (sorry, Tik-Tok®).

Morbidity – Harm short of death.

Morgue – Where dead bodies are stored before being transported to the funeral home.

Mortality – Death.

Mucociliary Escalator – The mechanism of mucus being slowly moved upwards through the respiratory tree by small hair (ciliary) cells beating rhythmically and in unison; prevents mucus accumulation in the airways.

Multi-Disciplinary Rounds – Performing patient rounds with staff from different disciplines, such as the nurse, pharmacist, respiratory therapist, and others, to provide more comprehensive care.

Multi-Drug-Resistant (MDR) Organism – A bacteria resistant to multiple antibiotics.

Multi-Organ Failure – Represents a domino effect where all the organs start to fail.

Myocardial Infarction (MI) – Heart attack; categorized into *non-ST elevation* (*N-STEMI*: muscle dying but not yet dead - bad) and *ST elevation* (*STEMI*: heart muscle death across the entire width – worse).

Myxedema Coma – A rare, life-threatening, extreme form of severely low thyroid hormones characterized by a slowed metabolic state, confusion or *coma*, low temperature, slow heart rate, and low blood pressure.

N

Nasal Cannula – Plastic tubing designed to deliver supplemental oxygen through the nose.

Nasogastric Tube (NG) – A soft plastic tube that goes down your nose and into the stomach; can be used to deliver nutrition and medication or can be set to suction.

Nebulizer – A device designed to aerosolize medication for breathing.

Nephrostomy Tube – Catheter inserted through the lower back/flank directly into the kidney to drain urine; may be used when the lower urinary track is blocked by a kidney stone or tumor.

Neuroleptic Malignant Syndrome – A very serious condition caused by antipsychotic medications characterized by high fever, muscle rigidity, and erratic blood pressure.

Neuromuscular Blocking Agents (NMBA) – Medications used to paralyze you to facilitate intubation or to allow you to breathe better while on a ventilator; also called *paralytics*.

Neutropenia – A dangerously low level of neutrophils, a type of white blood cell essential to fighting infections.

Night Float – The nighttime resident physician working in the hospital or the ICU.

Nil Per Os (NPO) or Nothing by Mouth – Indicates no eating, typically before a procedure or if you are too sick or confused to swallow.

Non-Invasive Positive Pressure Ventilation (NIPPV) – A ventilator that delivers air through a tight-fitting mask instead of an *endotracheal tube*; this support is used temporarily while the underlying problem (such as *COPD* or *CHF* exacerbation) can be corrected.

Non-rebreather Mask – A type of oxygen delivery mask that provides high concentrations of oxygen.

Non-small Cell Lung Cancer – A group of lung cancers that share characteristics.

Non-ST Elevation Myocardial Infarction (NSTEMI) – A type of heart attack typically treated medically.

Norepinephrine (Norepi) – A potent medication used to raise blood pressure.

Nosocomial – Healthcare-associated or hospital-acquired, generally referring to infections acquired at a health facility; may be caused by resistant organisms that require specialized antibiotics.

Nurse – A licensed health professional who takes care of you at the bedside, monitors you, and carries out your treatment orders.

Nurse Practitioner (NP) – Advanced practice registered nurse that can work independently and prescribe medications.

Nursing Home – A living environment with medical care provided by nurses and other staff on a continuous basis.

Nutritionist – A specialist who assesses your nutritional needs and how to best meet them.

O

Obesity Hypoventilation Syndrome (OHS) – Not breathing enough in your sleep due to being very overweight; leads to retention of carbon dioxide.

Obstructive Shock – Dangerously low blood pressure due to physical obstruction to blood flow into the heart, such as in a large *pulmonary embolism.*

Obstructive Sleep Apnea (OSA) – A condition where you stop breathing in your sleep due to airway obstruction (back of the throat collapsing); may lead to poor quality sleep and cardiovascular complications.

Obtunded – A reduced level of alertness and responsiveness.

Occupational Therapy – Therapy designed to assist with rehabilitating skills for everyday activities such as manipulating silverware, shoelaces, buttons, zippers, grooming, bathing, and more.

Open ICU – An ICU where you are cared for by a primary physician like a hospitalist or cardiologist, where an intensivist may serve as a consultant; any physician can write orders.

Organ Donation – The process of giving your organs to someone else.

Organ Procurement – The process of obtaining an organ for transplant; performed by a specialized team independent of the team taking care of you.

Orogastric Tube (OG) – A tube that goes through your mouth and into your stomach; usually used when you have an *endotracheal tube.*

Osteomyelitis – Infection of the bone requiring prolonged antibiotics

Outpatient – A patient not admitted to the hospital; a patient being seen in a clinic.

Oxygen – A life sustaining type of gas. Extra (*supplemental*) oxygen is provided when *room air* 21% is not enough; this saves your life if too low but is pro-inflammatory if too much is given.

Oxygen Saturation (Sp02) – The percentage of oxygen bound to *hemoglobin.* This can be determined by a *pulse oximeter* reading on the skin or nail surface.

P

Packed Red Blood Cells (PRBCs) – An essential blood product given to correct active bleeding and severe anemia.

Palliative Care – A branch of medicine focusing on symptom control; provided alongside other medical care. *End-of-life* and *hospice* care are part of palliative care.

Pan-consult – Getting a specialist for every organ; brings a lot of expertise but also a lot of cooks in the kitchen looking out for just their organ. Speaking of kitchen, may also refer to getting advice on the best pan for cooking.

Pancreatitis – Inflammation of the pancreas; commonly caused by obstructing gallstones and alcohol.

Paracentesis – A procedure that drains excess fluid from your abdominal cavity using ultrasound and a needle-based catheter device.

Paralytic – A medication that relaxes your muscles to the point of paralyzing you, also known as a *neuromuscular blocking agent* (*NMBA*).

Parathyroid Gland – Endocrine gland behind the thyroid that regulates calcium, phosphorus, and vitamin D.

Parenteral Nutrition – Nutrition provided directly into the vein.

Passey-Muir Valve (PMV) / Speech Valve – A one way valve attached to the tracheostomy tube that allows you to breathe in but closes as you breathe out thereby forcing the air up and through your vocal cords, allowing for speech.

Pathologist – A specialized physician who analyzes biopsy results and blood samples and performs autopsies.

Pathology – Abnormality.

Patient Controlled Analgesia (PCA) / Pain Pump – An *IV* with a button that the patient presses to give themselves pain medicine; can have a basal rate plus patient-controlled bolus with a lockout limit to prevent overdose.

Patient Safety – A part of the hospital administration dealing with patient safety concerns such as falls, hospital acquired infections, surgical errors, and so forth.

Percutaneous Endoscopic Gastrostomy (PEG) Tube – A feeding tube placed through the abdominal wall into the stomach.

Perfusionist – A technologist in charge of running an *ECMO* circuit.

Pericardial Drain – A catheter left in the space between the pericardial sac and the heart muscle to drain excess fluid.

Pericardial Sac – Lining surrounding the heart, also called the pericardium.

Pericardiocentesis – A procedure that removes excess fluid from the pericardial sac surrounding the heart using ultrasound and a special needle and catheter; if the catheter is left in, it is called a *pericardial drain.*

Pericarditis – Inflammation of the *pericardial sac;* may occur after viral infection.

Peripheral Edema – Swelling in the legs and arms, such as when fluid accumulates in the soft tissues commonly seen in heart failure, kidney or liver failure, and low protein states.

Peripherally Inserted Central Catheter (PICC) – A long catheter inserted through a smaller (peripheral) vein and passed through to a large (central) vein for longer term use, including at home; may also be used to draw blood.

Peripheral Parenteral Nutrition (PPN) – Partial nutrition through a regular or small vein.

Peritoneal Dialysis – A type of *dialysis* performed through liquid exchange in the abdomen.

Personal Protective Equipment (PPE) – Protective equipment worn to prevent contagious illness, including gloves, goggles, and masks.

Pharmacist – A medical professional with expertise in managing and dispensing medications, including following medication levels in the blood and adjusting the dosing; may also be responsible for mixing *TPN* and *PPN.*

Physical Therapy (PT) – Having to do with regaining muscle strength, ambulation, transfer abilities, joint flexibility, musculoskeletal and nerve pain rehabilitation, and more.

Physician Assistant (PA) – A licensed medical professional working under a physician to take care of patients; in the ICU often used to *round* on patients, complete charting, and perform procedures such as *lines,* under the direction of the *intensivist.*

Physician Assisted Suicide – A process where death is facilitated by a physician in the context of severe end-stage terminal illness; *euthanasia.*

Pig-Tail Catheter – A catheter with a curly end to help keep it in place; may be placed into the chest, abdomen, or other cavities to help decompress or drain abnormal collections of fluid or air.

Plasma – The liquid component of blood.

Plasma Exchanger – A machine similar to a *dialysis* machine that performs *plasmapheresis.*

Plasmapheresis – Similar to *dialysis,* a process that removes, treats, and replaces blood plasma to eliminate harmful antibodies or substances.

Pleural Effusion – A collection of fluid inside the chest cavity that compresses the lungs; common reasons are lung infection, heart failure, liver failure, and bleeding/trauma.

Pleurisy – Pain in the chest from inflammation of the lining of the lung or inside of the chest wall (pleura).

Pneumonia – Inflammation of the lungs commonly due to infection.

Pneumothorax – An intrusion of air into the chest cavity but outside the lung that collapses the lung and can be emergently dangerous necessitating placement of a *chest tube* to evacuate the air.

Pocket – A collection of fluid identified for drainage.

Podus Boot – A type of orthopedic boot designed to keep your foot flexed to prevent heel ulcers and foot drop.

Point of Care (POC) – A test that can be done at the bedside, like checking blood glucose levels.

Polycythemia – Too any red blood cells.

Portal Hypertension – Elevated pressures in the liver circulation typically due to *cirrhosis* or blood clots

Positive Emission Tomography (PET) Scan – A nuclear medicine scan designed to identify areas in your body with intense metabolic activity; risk stratifies a nodule or mass for cancer or infection ("lights up"), and to check for *metastatic disease*.

Pressors – A group of IV medications designed to artificially increase your blood pressure; IV versions of adrenaline.

Procalcitonin (Procal) – A blood test used as a marker of bacterial infections.

Prognosis – What we think is going to happen to you based on your medical situation.

Prophylaxis – Medications and devices meant to prevent complications; typical examples include stress stomach ulcer prophylaxis and *deep vein thrombosis* (*DVT*) prophylaxis.

Propofol – Generic name for *diprivan*, a potent IV sedative.

Proton Pump Inhibitor (PPI) – Strong medication used to decrease stomach acid and help prevent stomach ulcers including while critically ill.

Pulmonary Artery Catheter (PAC) / Swan Ganz Catheter (SGC) – A special venous catheter passed through the right side of the heart and into the circulation of the lungs; monitors the pressures inside the lung circulation and allows blood samples (*mixed venous oxygen saturation*).

Pulmonary Edema – Fluid accumulation or swelling in the lung causing difficulty breathing; often due to heart failure.

Pulmonary Embolism (PE) – A blood clot in the circulation of the lung; can be asymptomatic if small or deadly if large enough to occlude a significant amount of the blood supply to the lung.

Pulmonary Hypertension (PH) – Elevated blood pressure in the lung circulation; may cause significant shortness of breath and right-sided heart failure.

Pulse – The throbbing of an artery caused by pulsatile blood flow driven by the beating of the heart.

Pulse Oximeter – A device that detects the *pulse* and *oxygen saturation* when applied to the nail bed or skin.

Pyelonephritis – Infection of the kidneys that spread from the urinary tract; commonly presents as *costophrenic* (side of lower back) tenderness and may turn into *sepsis*.

Q

Quality Assurance – A hospital department that evaluates quality markers such as length of stay and nosocomial (hospital-acquired) infections and makes recommendations for improvement.

R

Radial Artery – main artery in your wrist supplying the hand; often used to measure *pulse*, and as a target for *arterial lines* and *arterial blood gas* samples.

Radiation Therapy – Type of cancer therapy using high energy beams (like X-rays).

Radiation Oncologist – Specialized radiologist with expertise in radiation therapy.

Rapid Infusion Protocol – A set of procedures to quickly infuse large amounts of *IV* fluids and blood products to treat *shock*, often with the use of a large IV and a mechanical rapid infuser; used in situations where significant blood loss has occurred.

Rapid Sequence Intubation (RSI) – A protocolized method for emergency *intubations* involving rapid administration of a sedative and *paralytic.*

Reciprocating Agreement – When a patient is transferred to another hospital, an agreement to transfer the patient back to the original hospital after the specialized care is provided.

Rectal Tube – A plastic tube inserted into the rectum to collect liquid stool so it doesn't keep messing the bed and breaking down your skin.

Renal Failure – Kidney failure.

Renal Replacement Therapy (RRT) – *Dialysis.*

Resuscitation – Saving you from the brink, as in *fluid resuscitation* where we give you lots of IV fluids to treat sepsis, or in *cardiopulmonary resuscitation* (*CPR*) where we compress your chest and provide other measures to try and save you.

Residency – A post-graduate (after graduating medical school) training program for physicians where they work under supervision to gain specialized expertise through hand-on learning.

Resident – A second (junior) or third (senior) year physician in a training program (*residency*).

Respiratory Failure – Having dangerously low levels of oxygen (*hypoxemic*) or high carbon dioxide (*hypercarbic*); further classified as acute or chronic.

Respiratory Therapy – Interventions pertaining to breathing like giving breathing treatments, running the ventilator, and performing lung function testing.

Restraints – Chemical (sedatives) or physical (mittens, wrist wraps, ankle wraps) ways to limit your movement to keep you safe (from pulling out lines and tubes or falling out of bed), and us when you are very agitated and confused.

Richmond Agitation-Sedation Scale (RASS) – Ranging from +4 (combative) to –4 (unarousable), a sedation scale used by your ICU nurse to titrate your sedative medications; a score of –1 (drowsy but sustained awakening) is the usual target when on a ventilator.

Right Heart Catheterization (RHC) – Placing a catheter through a vein into the right side of the heart to measure pressures in the lung circulation and identify *pulmonary hypertension.*

Risk Management – The part of the hospital administration concerned with getting sued.

Room Air (RA) – Refers to the percentage of oxygen in normal air, or 21% oxygen.

Rounds – Formal evaluation of your care including presentation of your case, review of data, physical exam, and plan formulation.

S

Sacral Decubitus Ulcer – A pressure sore at your tail bone; immobility, malnutrition, and failure to thrive put you at risk.

Salem Pump – A type of feeding tube.

Scleroderma – An autoimmune disease affecting many parts of the body including skin, kidneys (renal crisis), and joints.

Sedation – Using medications to help you relax

to different degrees, from taking the edge off to putting you into a medically induced coma.

Sedation Vacation – Holding or minimizing sedation to allow you to wake up and check your neurologic status and/or get you ready for *extubation*.

Senna – A natural laxative given to treat or prevent constipation while in the ICU; a common part of the bowel regimen.

Sensitivities – Referring to what specific antibiotics cultured bacteria are susceptible to.

Septic Shock – Dangerously low blood pressure triggered by infection and the immune over-response that follows.

Sepsis – An infection driven immune over-response that can cause shock and death.

Sequential Compression Devices (SCDs) – Massaging devices wrapped around your calves that inflate and deflate in sequence to keep the blood flowing and help prevent blood clots; also keeps you conveniently tied to the bed by your legs.

Serotonin Syndrome – A very dangerous syndrome caused by certain medications (certain antidepressants, triptans, opioids) that can include everything from diarrhea and anxiety to seizures and arrhythmias.

Sheath – Large IV catheter used to facilitate passage of other catheters and devices such as during cardiac catheterization.

Shock – Dangerously low blood pressure; commonly due to overwhelming infection (*septic*), acute blood loss (*hemorrhagic*), heart failure (*cardiogenic*), or *pulmonary embolus* (*obstructive*).

Sickle Cell Disease – A genetic disorder causing *red blood cells* to have an abnormal shape causing severe pain and low oxygen levels as they get stuck in small blood vessels.

Sigmoidoscopy – A procedure where a short scope is inserted through the anus to visualize the sigmoid, the lower part of the colon.

Sitter – A person who sits in your room to make sure you are safe and not pulling out your tubes and wires because you are confused.

Small Cell Lung Cancer – A type of lung cancer that tends to be aggressive and difficult to cure.

Sniffing Position – Extending your neck to help position your airway for intubation.

Social Worker – In the ICU, the professional who addresses complex social issues, facilitates communication, and obtains information such as the living will and healthcare proxy.

Sotalol – An antiarrhythmic used to slow down the heart rate.

Source Control – The concept of controlling the source of infection, such as removing an infected implant or catheter, or draining an abscess.

Speech Language Pathologist (SLP) – Speech therapist.

Speech Therapy – Therapy focused on swallowing and speech.

Speech Valve / Passey-Muir Valve (PMV) – A one way valve attached to the *tracheostomy* tube that allows you to breathe in but closes as you breathe out thereby forcing the air up and through your vocal cords, allowing for speech.

Spontaneous Bacterial Peritonitis (SBP) – Infection of the fluid in your abdomen (*ascites*), diagnosed by examining a sample of the abdominal fluid.

Spontaneous Breathing (Awakening) Trial (SBT/ SAT) – Breathing on your own through the ventilator to see if you are ready for extubation; occurs during a *sedation vacation*.

Spontaneous-Timed (ST) Mode – A mode in *non-invasive positive pressure ventilation* that has a back-up respiratory rate where pressurized air is pushed into you to help you breathe.

ST-Elevation Myocardial Infarction (STEMI) – A dangerous type of heart attack needing immediate intervention.

Stroke / Cerebrovascular Accident – An interruption of blood supply to the brain; most commonly, caused by blood clot (*thrombotic*), or bleeding (*hemorrhagic*).

Subcutaneous (SQ) – The area just under the skin; certain medications can be injected into this area.

Supportive Care – Refers to clinical interventions aimed at keeping you alive and comfortable while an illness runs its course.

Surgical Intensive Care Unit (SICU) – Where critically ill surgical patients are cared for.

Sustained Low-Efficiency Dialysis (SLED) – A type of sustained *dialysis* that is slow designed not to drop the blood pressure.

Swallow Evaluation – A bedside (done by the nurse) or more formal evaluation (by the speech therapist) to assess swallow ability; may include *fiberoptic endoscopic evaluation of swallowing* (*FEES*).

Swan Ganz Catheter (SGC) / Pulmonary Artery Catheter (PAC) - A special venous catheter passed through the right side of the heart and into the circulation of the lungs; monitors the pressures inside the lung circulation and allows blood samples (*mixed venous oxygen saturation*).

Systole – The part of the cardiac cycle where the heart muscles squeeze the blood forward.

Systolic Blood Pressure – The amount of force in your circulatory system when the main heart muscles squeeze; measured in mmHg, the top number of your blood pressure.

T

Tachycardia – An abnormally rapid heart rate.

TandemHeart® – An advanced heart therapy using a catheter and an external pump to push blood from the left atrium directly into the arterial system.

Targeted Temperature Management (TTM) – A protocol for reducing the body temperature (or preventing it from going too high) after a cardiac arrest designed to preserve brain function.

Teaching (Academic) Hospital – A hospital where teaching is a priority, staffed by medical students, residents, and sometimes fellows, who are working and learning at the same time.

Telemetry – A hospital unit where you wear a continuous heart monitor.

Tertiary Care Hospital – A hospital or medical facility providing advanced, highly specialized care for complex, severe, or rare health conditions.

Third Spacing – Fluid seeping out of your blood vessels and going into your soft tissues making you very swollen, as well as collecting in the abdominal cavity and chest; usually, a sign of too much fluid with kidney or heart failure, but also a marker of generalized inflammation and protein malnutrition.

Thoracentesis – A procedure to remove excess fluid from the chest cavity using ultrasound and a needle-based catheter system.

Thrombectomy – Removal of a blood clot by chemical or mechanical means.

Thrombocytopenia – Low platelet count; may predispose you to bleeding.

Thyroid Storm – A medical emergency caused by excessive production of thyroid hormones; may cause fever, confusion, high heart rate, vomiting, and diarrhea.

Total Parenteral Nutrition (TPN) – Full IV nutrition through a central or large vein.

Toxic Encephalopathy – Confusion due to being sick.

Trachea – Windpipe.

Tracheostomy – A hole created in the neck for insertion of a (tracheostomy) tube that provides direct access to the *trachea*; may be used for long term life support (*ventilation*).

Trade Name – A made up name of a drug given by the manufacturer who owns the trademark to sell the drug under that name; every medication has a trade name (sometimes multiple) and a single *generic* name.

Train of Four (TOF) – A way to determine effects of *paralytic* agents using electrical stimulation to a nerve followed by observation of muscle twitching; 1-2 is the usual goal.

Transfusion – Infusion of blood products.

Transfusion-Associated Circulatory Overload (TACO) – Having too much liquid volume in your system because of transfusion of blood products; can occur any day of the week.

Transfusion-Related Acute Lung Injury (TRALI) – A blood transfusion reaction that causes fluid to leak into the lungs resulting in *pulmonary edema*.

Translocation – Bacteria moving across the gut wall to cause infection in the blood stream or tissue; thought to occur during bowel wall damage and lower immune system function.

Transplant – Organ replacement.

Trauma Intensive Care Unit – Where critically ill trauma patients are cared for, such as after a motor vehicle accident, fall or burn injury.

Trendelenburg – A bed position where the whole bed is shifted with the foot of the bed up, like a seesaw; done during certain operations and during *central line* insertion into your neck veins.

Trialysis® Catheter – A special type of *dialysis* catheter that has an extra channel that can be used for IV therapy including during dialysis.

Triple Lumen Catheter (TLC) – A central *IV* line with three channels to be able to deliver multiple medications at once.

Tube 'em – Endotracheal intubation in preparation for putting you on a ventilator, as in "Tube 'em, partner."

Tube Feeds – Formula fed through a gastric tube.

Tumor – An abnormal growth of tissue, which may be benign or cancerous.

Tumor Lysis Syndrome – A constellation of chemical and electrolyte derangements caused by break down of tumor cells during cancer treatment; an oncologic emergency that can affect the kidneys, heart, and other organs.

Tunneled Catheter – A type of venous catheter that is passed under and parallel to the skin for several centimeters before going in the blood vessel; used for long–term venous access with less chance of displacement and infection.

U

Ultrafiltration – A very slow form of *dialysis* performed when the blood pressure is already dangerously low but fluid removal is required; does not replace hemodialysis.

Ultrasound – A harmless and extremely useful technology using sound waves to create a picture of different densities; used in many medical applications to help "see" inside the body.

Ureter – Tube transporting urine from the kidney to the bladder.

Urethra - Opening where urine comes out.

V

Varices – Abnormally dilated and swollen veins with high risk of rupture and bleeding.

Vasodilators – Medications used to make blood vessels relax to lower blood pressure.

Vasopressin – A potent medication used to increase very low blood pressure by constricting the blood vessels and promoting water reabsorption by the kidneys.

Vasovagal Reflex – An acute drop in blood pressure that can lead to fainting, sometimes due to pain, stress, or bearing down.

Veins – Blood vessels going towards the heart; a low pressure system with valves preventing backflow.

Veno-arterial (VA) ECMO - *Extra-corporeal membrane oxygenation* replacing the functions of the lungs and the heart.

Venovenous (VV) ECMO – *Extra-corporeal membrane oxygenation* replacing the function of the lungs.

Ventilation – The process of moving air into and out of the lungs, like you are doing right now (when you breathe).

Ventilation/Perfusion (V/Q) Scan – A nuclear medicine test used to detect blood clots in the lung circulation (*pulmonary emboli*); does not require intravenous contrast but does not show lung anatomy like a *CT* Chest.

Ventilator – A complex air compressor designed to deliver air through a mask or tube and help or replace your breathing.

Ventilator Facility – A medical facility for patients requiring long term *mechanical ventilation.*

Ventilator Mode – Collection of settings on a ventilator.

Ventilator Weaning – Refers to getting someone off the ventilator in a step-by-step fashion.

Venti-Mask / Venturi Mask – A type of oxygen mask that can be set to different percentages of inhaled oxygen.

Ventricle (brain) – A network of four cerebrospinal fluid-filled cavities in the brain.

Ventricle (heart) – The bottom chambers of the heart; right ventricle pumps blood into the lungs and the left ventricle pumps blood into the *aorta*/body circulation.

Ventricular Assist Device (VAD) – A mechanical device that helps pump blood through the heart when the heart is failing; may be a destination therapy (you can go home with certain VADs) or a bridge to heart transplant (used while waiting for a new heart).

Ventricular Fibrillation (V Fib) – A type of severe arrhythmia causing death where the ventricles of the heart go into "seizure" mode instead of pumping normally; can be reversed by electric shock (*defibrillation*) as seen in many movies and tv shows.

Versed® – Trade name for midazolam, a potent IV benzodiazepine type of sedative.

Veteran's Administration Medical Center (VAMC) – A hospital in the VA system catering to our country's veterans.

Virus – A category of microorganisms that include influenza (flu), respiratory syncytial virus (RSV), and COVID.

Vital Signs – Blood pressure, heart rate, oxygen level, respiratory rate, and temperature.

Voluntary Assisted Dying – *Euthanasia.*

W

Weaning Parameters – A set of respiratory maneuvers you perform while on a ventilator to see if you are strong enough to come off.

White Blood Cell (WBC) Count – The level of a group of cells in the blood that correlates with the activity of your immune system.

Wound Care – A set of interventions from topical medications to special bandages and even *wound vacuums* to address complex wounds; typically involves a wound care specialist.

Wound Vacuum – A device placed over large or complicated wounds that provides coverage and constant suction to protect the wound and remove excess fluid.

X

X-ray – A radiographic image that can show various pathologies (i.e. chest X-ray, abdominal X-ray, dental X-ray).

www.ingramcontent.com/pod-product-compliance
Lightning Source LLC
LaVergne TN
LVHW052256200926
848481LV00002B/379

* 9 7 9 8 9 9 4 6 2 2 6 0 5 *